The Patient's Guide to RSD

Essential Information for Patients with RSD

William Edward Ackerman III, MD

The Patient's Guide to RSD Essential Information for Patients with RSD

Copyright © 2010 by William Edward Ackerman III, MD

ISBN 145150604X

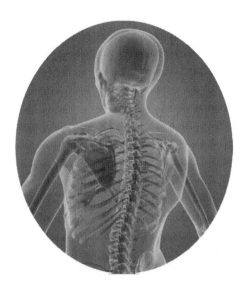

This book is dedicated to my loving wife Carrie, my dog, T Bone who recently passed away with cancer, my staff and to my patients whose questions concerning their RSD inspired the contents for this book.

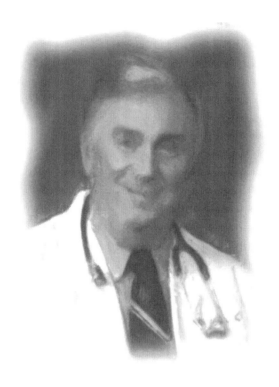

Dr. William Edward Ackerman III, MD is a clinician, a researcher, a scholar and an author who has done research and published his research on RSD/CRPS.

Acknowledgments

This book acknowledges patients suffering from RSD and their families who also suffer trying to comfort their family members tormented with horrific RSD related pain.

Foreword

Pain management is becoming an important and growing medical specialty. There is an attitude among individuals suffering from chronic pain that they are no longer willing to suffer pain in silence. Dramatic changes have been made with respect to the understanding of the anatomy any physiology of many painful entities over the past two decades. New drugs and other modalities are being introduced with increasing frequency. A pain patient needs to partner with his or her doctor. The reason for this book is to give a pain patient the basic information necessary to rationally discuss his or her RSD pain with their treating physician. Many primary care physicians as well as surgeons have no or minimal pain training. This book will enable a patient to derive basic pain management knowledge that may be helpful when he or she communicates with the pain management physician concerning RSD/CRPS treatments.

Table of Contents

1. An Overview of RSD/CRPS

Reflex sympathetic dystrophy (RSD) can be a devastating entity for you, especially if it is not diagnosed and treated within a timely fashion. Reflex sympathetic dystrophy usually affects one of your extremities (arms or legs) but also can affect your face. Reflex sympathetic dystrophy is now called the complex regional pain syndrome (CRPS). It can occur in children as well. In this chapter you will learn about your sympathetic nervous system and how it relates to complex regional pain syndromes. You will learn the differences between RSD and causalgia, another complex regional pain syndrome, but the pain conditions associated RSD will be discussed more in-depth. The three phases of RSD and its diagnosis will be discussed. You also will learn about your treatment options and current research findings. Reflex sympathetic dystrophy is serious, painful, and potentially disabling. Pain associated with this entity is throbbing, burning, or aching. You can have pain just to touch. You can have swelling of your extremity as well as either warmth or coldness depending on the phase of your RSD/CRPS and sweating. Your hair may grow faster on the extremity with RSD/CRPS at first, only to slow down as the disease progresses. Your extremity will sweat. It can turn color. The nails in your affected limb can grow faster on the extremity that suffers from reflex sympathetic dystrophy.

Reflex sympathetic dystrophy usually occurs following an injury. However, a heart attack or stroke can cause you to have reflex sympathetic dystrophy. It can also be seen in the knee as well as in the shoulder. In a study of reflex sympathetic dystrophy, 40 percent of the cases followed an injury to a muscle or a nerve. Simple bruises or sprains can trigger reflex sympathetic dystrophy. Fractures accounted for 25 percent of reflex sympathetic dystrophy cases. Twenty percent of the RSD/CRPS patients were postoperative on an arm or leg, whereas 12 percent occurred after a heart attack. Three percent occurred after a stroke. Approximately 37 percent of patients in the study had emotional disturbances at the time of the onset of the reflex sympathetic dystrophy.

It was once thought that reflex sympathetic dystrophy was a result of an emotional problem. However, studies have shown that many people do not suffer from emotional problems at the time of onset of reflex sympathetic dystrophy. Would you become anxious or depressed if your had constant severe pain that decreased your daily activity and disrupted your sleep? To prevent you from having permanent disability, treatment needs to be started immediately. Treatment usually consists of oral medications as well as injection therapy by an anesthesiologist using local anesthetics. Steroids may also be used effectively to treat RSD/CRPS. If your symptoms persist, sometimes you will need surgery to remove the offending nerves causing your pain.

As you can see, reflex sympathetic dystrophy can be potentially disabling. If you have any of the signs or symptoms of complex regional pain syndrome mentioned in this chapter, you should notify your doctor. Remember that early diagnosis and treatment can significantly improve your outcome. Further research in the exact cause of this disease and the appropriate treatment continues. If you have had reflex sympathetic dystrophy, it may have been called another condition. Only recently have scientists throughout the world come together at an International Association for the Study of Pain meeting. These scientists devised a term to describe reflex sympathetic dystrophy that is now called complex regional pain syndrome. At one time it was called post-traumatic sympathetic dystrophy, algodystrophy, Sudeck's atrophy, transient osteoporosis, and post-traumatic vasomotor syndrome. The shoulder/hand syndrome was also used to describe reflex sympathetic dystrophy following a heart attack or a stroke. If you sustained actual nerve damage, your reflex sympathetic dystrophy is called causalgia.

A previous definition of causalgia was referred to the syndrome associated with known nerve injury, whereas reflex sympathetic dystrophy included those patients whose pain and associated symptoms were followed by a variety of causes. Injury associated with causalgia was more severe, whereas that associated with RSD/CRPS was relatively minor. Now reflex sympathetic dystrophy is referred to as complex regional pain syndrome I, whereas causalgia is referred as complex regional pain syndrome II. Causes of both of these syndromes include fractures as well as dislocations. Reflex sympathetic dystrophy and causalgia were originally described by Dr. Mitchell, a neurologist during the Civil War. He noted that some soldiers who had injuries to their hands or feet developed a syndrome that consisted of burning pain, pain to touch over the skin of the injured extremity, shiny skin, and skin that had different colors consisting of either redness or a blue cyanotic color. Blue or cyanotic discoloration usually occurs when skin or other tissues do not get enough blood and oxygen. Dr. Mitchell also noted that the pain in the extremity was out of proportion to the injury. For example, if you sustained a sprain to your ankle, you would expect to have some pain. However, if you develop reflex sympathetic dystrophy, the pain is excruciating and unbearable. Mitchell noted the onset of reflex sympathetic dystrophy following gunshot wounds. The exact cause of reflex sympathetic dystrophy remains under investigation.

It was originally hypothesized that if your sympathetic nervous system became hyperactive, this hyperactivity was at least one of the causes of reflex sympathetic dystrophy. Your sympathetic nervous system is one component of your autonomic nervous system. The other component of your autonomic nervous system is called the parasympathetic nervous system. Your autonomic nervous system regulates your circulation and your breathing as well as your stomach and bladder functions. You have no control over your autonomic nervous system. This distinguishes it from your peripheral nervous system which is usually under your control. Because it is thought by some medical clinicians that your sympathetic nervous system can have some role in the onset of reflex sympathetic dystrophy, you must have a basic understanding of this system in order to understand reflex sympathetic dystrophy. Your sympathetic nervous system fibers emerge from your mid back part of your spinal cord. On the other hand your parasympathetic fibers come from your brain stem as well as your lower sacral areas. Your sympathetic nervous system sends sympathetic nerve fibers to the blood vessels in your head and neck as well as to your skin and muscles in your arms and legs. These fibers also go to your heart, your lungs, and your esophagus.

Furthermore, fibers can go to your stomach, pancreas, liver, gallbladder, and your intestines. Your kidneys, ureter, uterus, bladder, and prostate can all be affected. In your extremities, sympathetic fibers go to your blood vessels as well as your sweat glands and hair follicles. Remember that we said that your hands and feet can sweat profusely if you have reflex sympathetic dystrophy and the hair on your arms and legs can grow faster or fall out. Your sympathetic nerve fibers can restrict circulation in certain areas of your body.

Your sympathetic nervous system can also change the chemical environment of your muscle tissue as well as your other nervous system tissue and sensitive the small pain fibers in these different tissues. You must also realize that your sympathetic nervous system is linked to emotional states. Therefore, your sympathetic nervous system plays an important role in the psychological aspects of pain. Some-times if your doctor blocks your sympathetic nerve pathways, you can have some relief of your reflex sympathetic dystrophy. When you have an injury to your extremity, for example, you will have pain impulses that go to your spinal cord as well as your brain. The impulses that are going to your spinal cord and brain are initiated by pain fibers in your tissue. These pain fibers are both enhanced and inhibited at all levels of your brain and spinal cord. Your tissues produce pain-producing as well as pain-enhancing chemicals. This causes your nerves to transmit pain impulses onto your spinal cord and ultimately to your brain. However, in your spinal cord you have chemicals that can stop or attenuate the pain impulses.

You also have what are called descending pathways in your spinal cord, which are essentially nerves with chemicals that decrease the transmission of pain signals before they reach your brain. To modulate your pain, there must be checks and balances within your nervous system. Remember that pain is a warning to your brain that something is wrong at a particular place in your body. However, your body has normal mechanisms to lessen your pain. When you suffer from reflex sympathetic dystrophy, your pain-producing chemicals and nerves are much stronger than the aspects of your nervous system that are able to decrease the pain. Over time the part of your nervous system that decreases your pain becomes unable to function properly. At this time, your pain becomes overwhelming and disabling.

Chemical substances in your tissues activate your pain fibers. These chemicals cause your blood vessels to increase their diameter. When this happens, you will have warmth in your painful area as well as redness and increased temperature. As your blood vessels enlarge in diameter, you may also have swelling in your tissue. Chemicals such as acetychloline, potassium, and serotonin can stimulate pain in your tissues. However, when these chemicals are in your brain or spinal cord they do not cause pain. Histamine in your tissues can also be a chemical that can cause you to have pain. However, histamine is being used in creams to decrease your pain in your skin and muscles. Further studies have shown that the release of histamine into your spinal cord can decrease your pain as well. The mechanisms by which histamine either cause pain or help relieve pain remain to be studied and eluci-dated. Prostaglandins are also released if you have injury to your tissue. As mentioned previously, prostaglandins themselves do not produce pain; when they are around pain nerves, however, they sensitize these nerves to pain. Prostaglandins can intensify any inflammation that you may have and increase the action of bradykinin on your nerve endings. Substance P in your tissues can be a cause of significant pain. It is important for you to realize that there are many pain producing chemicals especially in reflex sympathetic dystrophy. You will note later in this chapter that different drugs are administered for the treatment of reflex sympathetic dystrophy.

The reason for this polypharmacy in the treatment of RSD/CRPS is that many chemicals combine to cause your pain associated with your reflex sympathetic dystrophy. If you have increased sweating associated with reflex sympathetic dystrophy, this implies that your sympathetic nervous system has become overactive. However, if your reflex sympathetic dystrophy persists over time, you will notice that your sweating in your hands or feet can significantly decrease. It is believed that with chronic reflex sympathetic dystrophy that the sympathetic reflexes do not remain active.

In 1916, a surgeon described that reflex sympathetic dystrophy pain could be relieved by surgically removing some of the sympathetic fibers that innervate the affected extremity. This surgeon also noted that patients who had his procedure had some pain relief and had decreased sweating and improvement in their skin color. This surgeon then thought that the sympathetic nervous system was involved in the etiology of reflex sympa-thetic dystrophy. In 1995, another doctor described another method using a scope for the removal of sympathetic nerve fibers that innervate your limb that has RSD/CRPS, and this has became a standard treatment for reflex sympathetic dystrophy. Over time the treatment of reflex sympa-thetic dystrophy included repetitive sympathetic blocks or removal of the sympathetic nerves, either surgically or by chemicals such as phenol. Sympathetic blocks involve placing a local anesthetic about the bundles of nerves which exist outside of your central nervous system. These nerve bundles which are called ganglia are in your neck as well as your lower back. The ganglion in your neck influences your arm pain while your ganglia in your lower back influences RSD/CRPS pain in your leg. These procedures for many years have been the standard treatment for the treatment of reflex sympathetic dystrophy. Finally, doctors who regularly treat reflex sympathetic dystrophy critically evaluated the effectiveness of these procedures. It is now known that temporary relief can occur with these procedures, but long-term results are poor. It is possible that these procedures have only survived time as a standard treatment for RSD/CRPS because of the lack of more effective therapy. Further-more, for years research on reflex sympathetic dystrophy was lacking because it was thought that this entity was mainly of a psychological origin.

Early descriptions of reflex sympathetic dystrophy included injuries without obvious nerve damage. Causalgia, on the other hand, was the description given to symptoms of reflex sympathetic dystrophy where a nerve had been actually injured, such as in a gunshot wound that was described by Dr. Mitchell during the Civil War. Sprains and strains can also be a cause of these syndromes as well as bursitis and tendonitis. Arthritis can also cause either reflex sympathetic dystrophy or causal-gia. If you are a female and have had a mastectomy, you may develop reflex sympathetic dystrophy. If one of the veins in your legs has been occluded, you may also develop reflex sympathetic dystrophy. After placement of a cast on your arms and legs, you may develop reflex sympathetic dystrophy and/or causalgia. Some individual have developed these syndromes following the onset of shingles. Head injuries and strokes can also cause you to have reflex sympathetic dystrophy or causalgia.

A rare but devastating form of reflex sympathetic dystrophy can occur after a tooth extraction (facial RSD/CRPS). Heart attacks can be associated with reflex sympathetic dystrophy of your upper arms. Painful reflex sympathetic dystrophy]like symptoms can occur around your perineum (the area between the anus and urinary outlet) following surgery around this area. Remember that sympathetic nerve fibers go to all parts of your body and, therefore, all parts of your body can be affected. The problem with reflex sympathetic dystrophy is that in many instances it is either over diagnosed or under diagnosed. A consensus conference, therefore, was held by doctors and scientists from all over the world. These individuals have compiled the diagnostic criteria for complex regional pain syndrome. The results of their meeting stated that complex regional pain syndrome describes a variety of painful conditions. The painful conditions must exceed the duration of the expected clinical course of the inciting event. For example, if you sustain an ankle sprain, your pain should be gone in several weeks. If your pain becomes severe and remains for several months, this suggests that you may have a complex regional pain syndrome. The problem with the two types of complex regional pain syndrome is that they can progress over time.

For you to be diagnosed with RSD/CRPS, you should have the following happen: An initiating traumatic event to your tissue, the onset of spontaneous pain as well as excruciating pain to touch as well as pain to a noxious stimulus that lasts longer than expected. Your pain must be global. For example, if you have injured your hand, you may have an injury to one of the nerves in your hand. For example, your ulnar nerve will give you pain or numbness in your last two fingers of your hand. This is the definition of a neuritis, which means inflammation of a nerve. This is not RSD/CRPS. RSD/CRPS means that the whole hand (global) is painful and not just in the distribution of one nerve. Evidence of swelling of your extremity, either an increase or a decrease in your skin blood flow as well as alterations in the color of your skin and sweating. The diagnosis of RSD/CRPS must be excluded by the existence of other conditions that could account for the degree of your pain and dysfunction. For example, arthritis and inflammation can give you pain that is similar to that of reflex sympathetic dystrophy.

For you to be diagnosed with causalgia, also known as complex regional pain syndrome II, you will have the above mentioned symptoms but you should also have a documented nerve injury. Further-more, for the diagnosis of both of these entities, you should have documented temperature changes noted on the skin over the area of your reflex sympathetic dystrophy. Remember that the diagnosis of CRPS cannot be made if you do not have pain. This is because CRPS is a pain syndrome by definition. Most of the time your pain will be of a burning nature. Your pain will develop after a traumatic event or after immobilization such as casting. Your pain will be on one side. Only rarely can reflex sympathetic dystrophy spread to another extremity. The onset of your symptoms usually occurs within a month from your surgery or trauma. You do not have reflex sympathetic dystrophy if you have anatomical, physiological, or psychological conditions that would cause your pain and dysfunction in your affected extremity. Remember that infection or arthritis are diseases that can mimic the symptoms of RSD/CRPS. These entities can cause you to have significant pain. If you have behavioral problems, your behavioral problems can be a cause of pain. If you become extremely anxious, you can have sweating associated that one normally sees in reflex sympathetic dystrophy. If you have complex regional pain syndrome, light touch or deep pressure should cause you pain. Cold applications to your skin can worsen your pain. Movement of your joints can also cause pain. You skin should be shiny. Your nails should grow faster on the side of the reflex sympathetic dystrophy. At first your hair will grow faster on the side of your reflex sympathetic dystrophy but eventually your hair pattern will decrease and you may even lose hair in this area. Tremors or spasms should be noted on the side of your reflex sympathetic dystrophy. If you have a complex regional pain syndrome, you should also have complaints of stiffness at the joints where your fingers meet your hand or where your toes meet your foot. Remember that the complex regional pain syndrome is usually over diagnosed. Unfortunately, some doctors will call shoddy surgery RSD/CRPS. This condition is rare. However, when it does occur, it must be treated immediately. If you have any of these symptoms mentioned in this chapter, notify your doctor.

Following surgery, reflex sympathetic dystrophy is a difficult entity to diagnose and treat. Studies on reflex sympathetic dystrophy, for example, following hand surgery can vary from less than 1 percent to 15 percent of all patients. As previously stated, reflex sympathetic dystrophy is often accompanied by dysfunction of your sympathetic nervous system, which results in changes in the blood flow to your skin of your affected limb. It was noted in 1946 that reflex sympathetic dystrophy needs to be diagnosed early because the treatment is more effective if you have an early diagnosis. In other words, early treatment positively affects your outcome. Blockade of your sympathetic nervous system is most effective for the treatment of your complex regional pain syndrome if it is performed within the first four to six weeks from the onset of your symptoms. These blocks become less effective the longer you wait to treat your complex regional pain syndrome. After surgery, the clinical diagnosis of RSD/CRPS is often delayed because RSD/CRPS can resemble normal postoperative states. If you have had hand surgery, for example, you can expect to have pain, swelling, and loss of function as well as the other symptoms associated with reflex sympathetic dystrophy. However, these symptoms should be gone by six weeks.

At one time, it was thought that a three-phase bone scan was useful for the diagnosis of complex regional pain syndrome. Studies were done as early as 1981. Individuals also used the three-phase bone scan for monitoring the progress of RSD/CRPS. This imagery is related to the distribution of a radioactive isotope throughout the body, and a nuclear medicine doctor will note the distribution of this radioactive isotope in the affected extremity. The distribution of the radioactive isotope is dependent upon blood flow as well as the activity of the bone. The problem with this test is that it has not been shown to be as good as previously assumed. Furthermore, if your three-phase bone scan is negative, this does not mean that you do not have reflex sympathetic dystrophy.

A study in 2001 found that the three-phase bone scan was positive in only 53 percent of the individuals studied. Furthermore, it was published in 1999 that the three-phase bone scan is of little value in monitoring the course of the treatment of your complex regional pain syndrome. A three-phase bone scan may be effective for staging the early or late forms of RSD/CRPS. Magnetic resonance imaging (MRI) can aid in the diagnosis of RSD/CRPS by identifying swelling in the center of your bone. This bone marrow edema is characteristic of complex regional pain syndrome. This study is more reliable than a three-phase bone scanning or plain x-ray exams. In 2002, it was reported in a pain medical journal that skin temperature differences in the arms and legs are extremely useful for the diagnosis of complex regional pain syndrome. Contact and infrared thermography have both been recommended for the diagnosis of reflex sympathetic dystrophy, but the problem with thermography is that it can be influenced not only by skin blood flow but also by the temperature of the room environ-ment as well as by your muscle and your deep tissue metabolism.

A new method called laser Doppler imaging has been shown to be effective for the diagnosis of complex regional pain syndrome. This is a new entity and is not readily available in most medical centers or doctors' offices. It is a noninvasive procedure that takes no more than 10 minutes for your evaluation. It measures your skin blood flow. This laser Doppler is important because the results of this study is influenced by your superficial blood flow. Your superficial blood flow is under the control of your autonomic nervous system. Other studies are being developed, which include plethsmography and capillaroscopy. Another device to evaluate reflex sympathetic dystrophy is called the quantitative pseudomotor axon test. This test is time-consuming and is currently available only in several academic centers. However, the results of this test are accurate.

There are different phases of reflex sympathetic dystrophy. A test that measures all three of these phases is necessary. The only one to date that will detect all three phases is the laser Doppler device. After you have sustained an injury to your extremity, the blood vessels to your extremity become bigger. This allows more blood flow to go to your extremity. Your hand or foot will, therefore, feel warm and may appear to be red. This phase usually occurs within the first month of your injury. A three-phase bone scan at this time will demonstrate increased isotope activity in your extremity, which indicates phase I reflex sympathetic dystrophy.

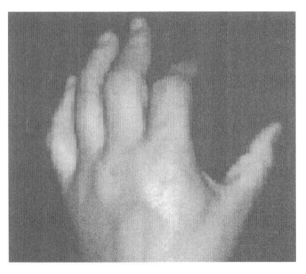

Figure 1. Phase I, RSD/CRPS. Note the swollen hand and fingers.

As your RSD/CRPS progresses, the blood vessels to your extremity will decrease in diameter. They go from the enlarged diameter to a normal appearing diameter. This is phase II CRPS/RSD. A three-phase bone scan will, therefore, appear normal at this time. A laser Doppler study, on the other hand, will reveal an abnormality of your sympathetic nervous system. You will have some swelling as well at this time and global pain about your extremity and sweating of your extremity as your sympathetic nervous system becomes overactive. This phase can progress on to Phase III RSD/CRPS. During this phase, your blood vessels become extremely small and you have decreased blood flow to your hand, foot, or your affected extremity. This will cause your skin to become cold. By this time, you will notice that your skin has become shiny and that the sweating in your hand or foot may have increased. A three-phase bone scan at this time can detect a significant decrease in your blood flow to your extremity. Your treating doctor should try and prevent you from progressing through these phases.

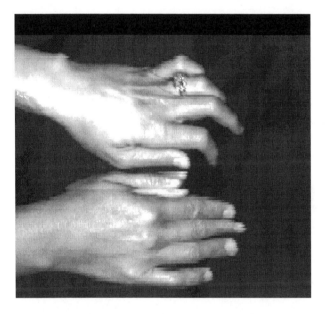

Figure 2. Phase III, RSD/CRPS of the left hand. Note the shrinkage of the muscles of the left hand when compared to the patient's right hand. The fingers of the left hand are in a flexed position as a result of the muscle shrinkage(atrophy).

As stated previously, an early diagnosis and treatment will prevent this progression to the worst phase. After you have reached phase three of reflex sympathetic dystrophy, the disease is irreversible. The success rate for phase I is extremely high, which does decrease as you progress to phase II. This is the reason why you should keep an accurate and thorough pain diary. Your symptoms of your pain will provide some suggestion to your doctor as to what phase of reflex sympathetic dystrophy that you are in. In all the phases, you will need an occupational therapy evaluation to attempt to desensitize the pain in your skin and to preserve normal range of motion in your hand, foot, arm, leg, and so on. A study from the Netherlands published in 1993 noted symptoms and signs of complex regional pain syndrome. Pain was noted in 84 percent of individuals longer than 12 months. Ninety-one percent had temperature differences in their extremities after 12 months. Recurrence with exercise was noted in 97 percent of patients. Fifty-five percent continued to have swelling after 12 months. Muscle spasms were noted in 42 percent of individuals. Sweating was noted in 40 percent of patients. Nail growth continued in 52 percent of individuals, whereas hair patterns were present in only 35 percent of patients.

Be aware that on rare occasions RSD/CRPS can spread into more than one extremity. This observation suggests that an individual may have a predisposition to develop RSD/CRPS. If you have chronic RSD/CRPS, you can have skin infections associated with persistent swelling of your skin as well as blood vessels that can spontaneously rupture. You may have a change in skin pigmentation and your fingernails or toenails on the affected extremity can become clubbed. The frequency of reflex sympathetic dystrophy shows a peak of the incidence of this entity around 50 years of age. However, you must be aware that both children and elderly individuals can develop RSD/CRPS.

The distribution of RSD/CRPS between men and women is almost equal for individuals younger than 50 years of age. However, for those over 50 years of age there is a predominance of reflex sympathetic dystrophy noted in women. Even though some investigators have questioned the existence of the sympathetic nervous system's influence on the pain associated with reflex sympathetic dystrophy, there is clinical evidence that this influence does actually exist. This led investigators to describe two types of pain. One is sympathetically maintained pain and is pain associated with chemicals released by the sympathetic nervous system. The other type of pain is sympathetically independent pain, which is not associated with the chemicals liberated by the sympathetic nervous system into the bloodstream. Other types of pains can be responsive to sympathetic blockade. This type of blockade with a local anesthetic can even decrease pain associated with peripheral nerves. Sympathetically maintained pain usually has a decrease in your pain component following a sympathetic block. Sympathetically maintained pain can be seen in other entities besides reflex sympathetic dystrophy. It may be seen in neuropathies, phantom limb pain, and shingles as well as neuralgias.

The onset of reflex sympathetic dystrophy can occur at any time following a traumatic event. It was thought at one time that RSD/CRPS could occur without any trauma. This is no longer thought to be true. There is a case report of reflex sympathetic dystrophy beginning one year after a fracture occurred. Exact causes of reflex sympathetic dystrophy continue to be studied. As stated previously, it is thought that there is a sympathetic nervous system component that causes you to have pain when you develop reflex sympathetic dystrophy. Your nerve ending develop an abnormal sensitivity to the chemicals that are liberated by your sympathetic nerve fibers. If you have had a nerve injury, your nerve will attempt to regrow and will sprout small sensory pain fibers. Sometimes as your nerves attempt to grow together, the area where they come together can be extremely painful. Where the nerve endings come together can cause an extremely painful area called a neuroma. This neuroma is sensitive to the chemicals released by your sympathetic nervous system.

Most medical investigators report that over time the sympathetic nervous system becomes less involved in the maintenance of reflex sympathetic dystrophy syndrome. As mentioned earlier in this chapter, you can have reflex sympathetic dystrophy that does not involve a nerve injury. In 1996, it was reported that the peripheral nervous system as well as the central nervous system is involved in the progression of RSD/CRPS. With this type of pain, your pain receptors may be stimulated by both sympathetic nervous system biochemicals such as norepinephrine or through the release of prostaglandins. Prostaglandins will sensitize your nerve endings to other substances that are in your tissues. The prevalent theory is that pain associated with reflex sympathetic dystrophy is mediated by prostaglandins.

Because many individuals have no decrease in their pain when they have sympathetic blocks in both reflex sympathetic dystrophy and causalgia, many investigators question the existence of any sympathetic involvement in these pain syndromes. In 1995, it was proposed that inflammation with the release of prostaglandins function was the cause of pain in both RSD/CRPS and causalgia. Furthermore, evidence indicates an inflammatory basis for the loss of bone mass that occurs in reflex sympathetic dystrophy. More recent studies have determined that the COX-2 enzyme may be responsible for the pain associated with reflex sympathetic dystrophy. This is the reason why many doctors today treat reflex sympathetic dystrophy with the new COX-2-inhibiting drugs such as Celebrex. Furthermore, there may be an interaction between COX-2 enzyme and stimulation of the sympathetic nervous system.

Even though your injury usually occurs in your arms or legs, there can be distorted information processing within your spinal cord. In other words, changes in your spinal cord can occur secondary to your nerve injury in your arms or legs. Small inhibitory nerves in your spinal cord, called internuncial neurons, may be ineffective if you develop reflex sympathetic dystrophy. In addition to your central nervous system (composed of your brain and spinal cord) as well as your peripheral nervous system, which is composed of nerves outside of your brain and spinal cord, you also have a sympathetic nervous system. Studies have shown that females are more vulnerable to sympathetically mediated pain than males. The chemicals that are involved that cause you to have reflex sympathetic dystrophy are potentially affected by your sex hormones. It is believed that your hormone status at the time of your trauma is important for the development of the pain associated with reflex sympathetic dystrophy.

The effects of reflex sympathetic dystrophy on the central processing in your central nervous system may be the basis for the spread of reflex sympathetic dystrophy to your other extremities. Many recommendations for the treatment of reflex sympathetic dystrophy and causalgia exist. Because there are so many different treatments proposed, you should be aware that no single treatment is superior to the others. Remember that no treatment for complex regional pain syndrome is consistently successful. It is known that early recognition and active treatment of the complex regional pain syndrome improves your outcome. For example, injec-tions of local anesthetics about your sympathetic nervous system can alleviate your symptoms of reflex sympathetic dystrophy long term. These types of injections must be done early in the onset of your symptoms of reflex sympathetic dystrophy. The injections can be done in your stellate ganglion, which provides sympathetic fibers to your arms, or the injections can be done in the lumbar sympathetic ganglion, which supplies sympathetic fibers to your legs. Because disuse of your extremities can contribute to the onset of reflex sympathetic dystrophy, your doctor will institute occupational therapy for you. This type of therapy emphasizes range of motion. As stated previously, the new COX-2-inhibiting drugs can be helpful in decreasing your pain associated with complex regional pain syndrome. A Clonidine patch can be used to decrease your pain. This patch is usually used to treat high blood pressure. However, the patch does decrease the sympathetic nervous system chemicals that can be released if you have reflex sympathetic dystrophy. The patch is usually worn for one week before it is changed.

Steroids administered by mouth have been shown to be effective for the treatment of reflex sympathetic dystrophy. Steroids will decrease inflammation caused by prostaglandins. If your pain is severe, your doctor will probably prescribe a narcotic drug for you. Depending on the severity of your pain, your doctor will prescribe a mild narcotic such as Darvocet or a stronger narcotic such as Methadone. Anticonvulsive medications can be helpful in decreasing your pain. Gabapentin (Neurontin) is frequently used now for the treatment of pain associated with your complex regional pain syndrome medications administered into your spinal fluid can also help decrease your pain. Sometimes a morphine pump, which sends a narcotic into your spinal fluid, needs to be implanted to control your RSD/CRPS pain. Clonidine, which is frequently administered by a patch over your skin, can also be administered into your epidural space for the control of your pain as well. Antidepressant medication such as amitriptyline has also been shown to be effective in the management of pain associated with reflex sympathetic dystrophy and causalgia. Amitriptyline increases certain chemicals in your central nervous system that are helpful in decreasing the amount of pain that reaches your brain. Implantation of a wire attached to a battery into your epidural space can also provide you with significant pain relief. This apparatus is called a dorsal column stimulator. Psychological intervention is also helpful; because of the severity of the pain associated with reflex sympathetic dystrophy, you can develop fear, anxiety, and depression. Psychological intervention including the use of biofeedback and sometimes hypnosis can success-fully be used to treat your pain.

Early in your symptoms of RSD/CRPS, your doctor can inject local anesthetic near your ganglion to relieve pain in your sympathetic nervous system. Local long-acting anesthetic injections may be needed in your areas of discomfort to help relieve your pain. Steroids can help reduce inflammation caused by prostaglandins. Your doctor may prescribe narcotic medications such as morphine and Clonidine to help control your pain. Antidepressant medications prescribed by your doctor can increase certain chemicals in your central nervous system that are helpful in reducing the amount of pain impulses that reach your brain. Some RSD/CRPS patients may require psychological therapy, such as biofeedback, to help treat the fear, anxiety, and depression they may feel because of their painful condition.

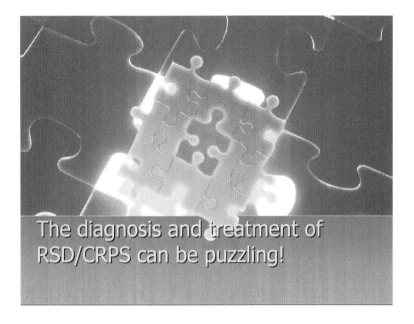

The diagnosis and treatment of RSD/CRPS can be puzzling!

It may be concluded that RSD/CRPS can be a difficult entity to diagnose and treat. Remember that an early diagnosis with the imitation of treatment in a timely fashion is the key to the successful resolution of CRPS/RSD.

2. Pain Anatomy

The word "pain" is derived from the Latin word poena that means punishment. St. Augustine wrote in the 5th century that all diseases afflicting Christians were derived from demons. Ancient tribal concepts of pain were based on beliefs that evil spirits were sent as punishment from their gods to invade one's body and cause severe pain. In the book of Genesis, Eve was condemned to pain during childbirth as a result of her encounter with the devil in the Garden of Eden. It has been reported that a shaman could suck an evil spirit from a wound to decrease one's pain. The ancient Greeks such as Aristotle were the first individuals who believed that pain was derived from various nerves in the body. The exact cause of pain was unknown to them. Unfortunately, not unlike ancient times, the diagnosis and treatment of many chronic painful conditions today remains mostly guesswork. Pain medicine is for the most part subjectively based, because pain is a subjective symptom while other medical specialties are based upon objective medical evidence. Pain in general is not bad. Pain is a protective mechanism that warns you that your body has something wrong at some location. The sensation of pain tells you to stop activity or to at least slow down your activity. For example if you sprain your ankle, your pain is a warning for you not to put weight on that leg. The International Association for the Study of Pain defines pain as" an unpleasant sensory and emotional experience associated with tissue injury as a result of trauma (e.g. bone fracture) or disease (e.g. cancer, shingles).

Pain has psychological effects in some instances especially when pain is severe. Pain may cause anxiety and depression. Acute pain is associated with injury, bone fractures, surgery or sprains and strains. Once these entities have healed sometimes, the pain continues. Arthritis is another example of chronic pain. Arthritic pain is caused by continuous joint destruction. However, once the pain becomes chronic, your pain it becomes a problem. Not only does pain become a personal problem but pain can become a social problem with creation of family problems, loss of self esteem and lost wages. Fibromyalgia patients have alterations in CNS anatomy, physiology, and chemistry that potentially contribute to the symptoms experienced by these patients

The purpose of this chapter is to present you with the basic anatomy and physiology of painful sensations. Pain impulses are in essence, electrical signals that travel from various areas of your body such as the extremities, heart, appendix etc. to the spinal cord and eventually reach the brain where the pain signals are processed like data in a computer. The brain is like a computer hard drive, which stores painful experiences that ultimately results in the suffering associated with chronic pain. Pain is produced by unpleasant stimuli to nerve endings throughout the body which include chemical, extreme heat cold and mechanical injury. These nerve endings are silent until mechanical, heat or cold injures tissue. In order to experience pain we need these pain receptors and the nerve fibers that transmit pain to the spinal cord and then to the brain.

Nerves, which conduct pain impulses to the spinal cord, are composed of neurons (nerve cells) that make up nerve fibers that form neurons. Two common pain fibers are the C fibers and the A-delta fibers. A-delta fibers conduct fast onset sharp pain impulses. The C fibers conduct slow onset dull, aching or burning pain. If you hit your finger with a hammer, you will experience a sudden pain response followed by a dull pain response. Other types of fibers that transmit touch and vibration exist do not cause pain in most instances. However, these fibers can become hypersensitive and may contribute to your total pain experience. A neuron is an electrically excitable cell in the nervous system that processes and transmits information. Neurons are the significant core components of your brain and spinal cord as well as your peripheral nerves.

Neurons are typically composed of a cell body, a dendrite and an axon. Neurons receive input from dendrites and transmit output via the axon. Neurons are the building blocks of nerves. In other words, multitudes of neurons are necessary to form a nerve. Nerves that exist outside of your central nervous system are called a ganglion. Your stellate ganglion in your neck is an example. An injection into this ganglion may relieve pain associated with Reflex Sympathetic Dystrophy (now called Complex Regional Pain Syndrome). Various ganglia may form a plexus. An example of a plexus is your celiac plexus. Sometimes this plexus is blocked with numbing medicine or phenol or alcohol to relieve severe abdominal pain.

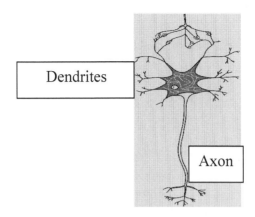

Figure 1. A nerve is composed of neurons. A neuron has one axon that takes nerve signals away from the neuron. The long end of the axon communicates with multiple dendrites.

Action potentials generated by the neuron initiate pain signals. If your skin is pinched a mechanical pain receptor begins and action potential. An action potential begins after a depolarization (a change in the electrical activity within the neuron) such that it could cause a membrane transitory modification, turning prevalently permeable to sodium ions more than to potassium ions. Sodium permeability can cause an action potential.

Neuropathy generates a local accumulation of sodium channels, with a consequent increase of density. This remodel seems to be the basis of neurohyperexcitability. Calcium channels have also an important role in cell function. Intracellular calcium increase contributes to depolarization processes, through kinase and determines the phosphorylation of membrane proteins that can make powerful the efficacy of the channels themselves. Following an acute injury, AMPA receptors are stimulated which cause sharp pain. Receptors (areas in the body where biochemicals or drugs attach) are present in the spinal cord are called NMDA (N-methyl-D-aspartate) receptors and cause chronic pain.. When these NMDA receptors are stimulated, pain becomes more severe and this severe pain is maintained which implies that the pain does not decrease. The brain is responsible for the suffering associated with pain. Pain results in bodily responses especially with respect to the cardiovascular system (heart rate increases, blood pressure increases, renal arteries constrict etc). When pain is severe, the brain can cause the body to increase both the heart rate and blood pressure. Severe pain can also result in profuse sweating as well as nausea and vomiting. There are different types of nerve endings throughout the body. The pain nerve endings become hyper excitable when stimulated by injury, inflammation or a tumor. Occasionally the nerve endings remain irritable even after the painful stimulus has been removed. Pain signals from areas in the body reach the brain by four processes (transduction, transmission, modulation and perception).

Axons carry pain fibers away from your neuron and direct them to the dendrites of the next neuron until they terminate in your brain or spinal cord. Remember that the axons and dendrites do not touch. They form synapses or clefts between the axon and dendrite. The synapse has chemicals in the axon nerve ending. These chemicals allow communication between the neurons. Drugs are chemicals that can interrupt the communication between the neurons. Hypnosis and biofeedback can disrupt pain signal transmission. Injections can also inhibit transmission of pain signals from your arms or legs to your brain.

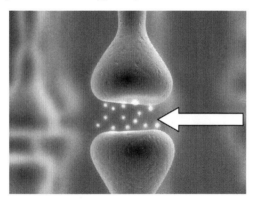

Figure 2. Chemicals are transferred between nerve endings (synapses) which cause transmission of pain signals. Pain signals may be blocked if the chemicals are inhibited from passing from one nerve to another.

You need to understand that pain signals cross to the opposite side from the injury and therefore travel to the opposite side of your brain. Figure 3 demonstrates this concept. The following illustration demonstrates by the arrows that pain signals enter the back of your spinal cord. They cross over to the other side. The pain impulses will then proceed upwards to go to your brain. It is important to know that pain signals can be dampened by structures and chemicals that exist in your spinal cord. Pain signals as mentioned previously are transmitted from the site of injury as action potentials. Electrical and/or chemical activity between the neuron dendrites and axons propagate the axon potentials.

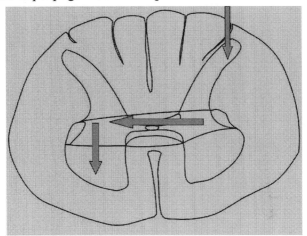

Figure 3. Cross section of the spinal cord that demonstrates the site (at the top of the diagram) where pain signals enter your spinal cord, then cross to the other side of your spinal cord and proceed upward to your brain. Pain on your right side goes to the left side of your brain.

It is important to understand the following processes in order to understand how your pain can be treated effectively. Transduction is a process where electrical signals originate in the nerve endings throughout your body. These impulses are chemically, mechanically and/or thermally mediated and transmitted to your spinal cord where they can be modulated and then sent to your brain. Tissue injury or disease (including arthritis) cause the body to release biochemicals called prostaglandins. Prostaglandins themselves do not cause pain. Prostaglandins do however sensitize pain receptors to other chemicals in the body, which facilitate the transmission of pain impulses. Nonsteroidal drugs like ibuprofen decrease the number of prostaglandins produced in your body and may in a decrease in your pain perception. Topical creams such as Ben Gay can decrease the process of transduction at the nerve endings.

Transmission is a process where pain signals are transported to the spinal cord. Nerves in body tissues transmit impulses to the spinal cord. Nerve blocks with anesthetics like Novicaine can interrupt the transmission of pain impulses to the spinal cord. Once pain impulses reach the spinal cord they are modulated or changed by chemicals and nerves that inhibit or lessen the number of pain impulses from going up the spinal cord to your brain. Fibers called internuncial fibers are present within the spinal cord that can decrease pain transmission. The brain can send impulses back to these pain control fibers within the spinal cord to decrease the number of impulses that reach the pain perception center of the brain. This is the basis of hypnosis. Severe pain however, overwhelms the nerve fibers and hypnosis essentially becomes ineffective. Most pain impulses cross over into the opposite side of the spinal cord from where they entered the spinal cord. The spinal cord acts like a transformer to intensify or decrease the intensity of pain impulses. Narcotics and anticonvulsants can modulate pain impulses within the spinal cord. Finally, pain impulses reach the brain where you perceive pain. Be aware that pain signals enter the posterior part of your spinal cord (figure 1) and then cross to the other side and travel upwards to the pain processing of your brain.

Narcotics can "numb" your brain to decrease the effects of the pain impulses on your brain by decreasing the intensity of these impulses. Higher brain centers determine how we respond to a painful stimulus. This explains why an individual can respond differently to a painful stimulus from other individuals (eg. "cry baby, whiner, vs macho man etc.). A chapter describing the anatomy and physiology of pain is not complete without an explanation of the Gate Control Theory of pain. Melzak and Wall described this theory in 1965. Different types of nerve fibers (both pain and non pain fibers) enter the spinal cord at the same time. Non-pain fibers essentially dilute out the number of pain impulses that enter the spinal cord. An example of the Gate Control Theory is given by the following analogy. If you can imagine severe pain impulses represented by of multiple black balls going down a sink (analogy to spinal cord). If one adds multiple white balls (neutral non-pain transmitting entities), the number of black balls (pain impulses) is diluted. Therefore less severe pain impulses reach the spinal cord and the brain. The white balls are non-pain balls and can close the gate (drain) to the number of black balls that go down the sink. To open the gate to more pain impulses, one only needs to decrease the number of white balls going to the hole in the sink. At this time, there are more black balls (pain impulses) available. The gate is now open. As you can see, pain perception in the human body is com-plex. Because there are many different chemical transmitters and anat-omic structures that contribute to chronic pain syndromes, each patient's treatment must be individualized. This is where the art of pain medicine is separated from pure science.

In order to understand pain transmission concepts, you must first become familiar with several biochemicals that are stored in your body that affect your pain signals. In order for you to hurt, pain-producing chemicals in your body tissue must stimulate pain fibers (Alpha-delta and C fibers). In general, the greater the tissue trauma, the more pain transmitting chemicals are produced and the worse the pain. In medical terminology, a stimulus (pin prick) produces a response (pain perception). When a stimulus such as heat produces, tissue injury chemicals are released at the site of nerve injury, which cause pain fibers to become hyperactive. These chemicals include bradykinin, histamine, substance p, acetylcholine, serotonin and histamine. These chemicals act at the nerve endings and ultimately travel to the spinal cord and brain.

The nerves that conduct pain go to the spinal cord that allows pain signals to ultimately reach the brain. Areas of your body that have many pain receptors include the skin, the outer aspect of bone called the periosteum, ligaments, joints, teeth and gums and the cornea of the eye. Muscle also contains pain fibers but not as many per square meter (a measure of area) as the previously mentioned structures. Where the nerves from your body enter your spinal cord, aspartic and glutamic acid are produced. These acids increase pain impulse generation. NMDA may also be produced. GABA (gamma-aminobutyric acid) in the spinal cord on the other hand, decreases the number of pain impulses that reach the brain. GABA inhibits pain impulse transmission. Norepinepherine and serotonin are two more chemicals in the spinal cord which attenuate the number of pain impulses which reach your brain. The brain and spinal cord regulate pain by the production of naturally occurring narcotic-like substances that decrease pain transmission in specific areas of the brain. These narcotic-like drugs are called enkephalins, dynorphins and beta-endorphins. Some of these substances also decrease pain transmission in the spinal cord. Enkephalins are located in areas of the brain related to pain modulation.

Enkephalins inhibit pain at the spinal cord level. Enkephalins bind to narcotic receptors. When the narcotic receptors are activated, they inhibit pain signals. Dynorphins exist in both the brain and spinal cord but are more prevalent in the brain. Like enkephalins these substances bind to narcotic receptors in the brain and spinal cord. Pain impulses that enter your spinal cord cross over to the other side and then progress upward to your brain. The natural beta-endorphins in your body exhibit morphine-like activity. They work like morphine to decrease your pain. Following injury or stress these endorphins are released into the blood stream. The effects of beta-endorphins are similar to morphine. Beta-endorphins like narcotics can cause respiratory depression, constipation, euphoria, toler-ance and physical dependence. The exact biochemical actions of all of the substances mentioned are complex. For a more detailed explanation of the actions of these substances one should consult a pain medicine text-book. The purpose of this chapter is to emphasize the multiple substances that can generate the transmission of pain signals. This is furthermore the reason why there are so many medications available for the management of your pain. This is also the reason why your physician may prescribe multiple medications for the management of your chronic pain.

With respect to tissue and nerve ending biochemicals, neurotransmitters and pain transduction, your physician may recommend a skin (topical) cream to decrease the transmission of pain signals to your brain. Red pepper cream decreases the pain generator called substance P. An exam-ple is Zostrix cream. Menthol containing creams (Ben Gay®) also decrease pain over muscles and joints. Non-steroidal anti-inflammatory drugs (NSAIDS) decrease the production of prostaglandin that can sensi-tize your body to pain mediators. Examples include Advil and Celebrex. Remember that prostaglandins sensitize pain nerve endings to pain producing tissue chemicals. Antidepressant drugs like Elavil or Prozac decrease pain by increasing norepinephrine and serotonin in the spinal cord. As previously mentioned, these two substances decrease the number of pain impulses that reach the pain perception areas of the brain. Anti-convulsant drugs like Gabitril (tiagabine) in some instances affect GABA levels in your spinal cord and by enhancing GABA blood levels decreases the number of pain signals in your spinal cord that can go to your brain. Narcotic drugs also decrease pain impulse conduction in both the spinal cord and brain. Injections of numbing medicine (local anesthetics with steroids) can decrease pain in muscle and nerves in the arms, legs and the trunk of the body. Epidural steroid injections can decrease pain in nerves that are buried deep within the spine. As you see there are multiple biochemical sources of pain and in many instances your physician may elect to prescribe multiple medications with good reason. Remember that each of these medications can have side effects that will be discussed in a later chapter.

There is an area of your brain that represents an area where you process pain signals. This area detects tissue injury and is a protective mechanism to alert you that something is wrong. A burn of the palm of your hand alerts your brain that tissue injury is occurring and initiates a reflex in your spinal cord to have you immediately remove your hand from the hot object. Without pain interpretation in your brain, you could sustain multiple bodily trauma and have no knowledge of its occurrence. The different dimensions of pain perception have been shown to depend on different areas of your brain. In contrast, much less is known about the neural basis of pathological chronic pain. Patients may report combinations of spontaneous pain and allodynia/hyperalgesia-abnormal pain evoked by stimuli that normally induce no/little sensation of pain. Modern neuroimaging methods (positron emission tomography (PET) and functional MRI (fMRI)) have been used to determine whether different neuropathic pain symptoms involve similar brain structures. PET studies have suggested that spontaneous neuropathic pain is associated principally with changes in thalamic activity and the medial pain system, which is preferentially involved in the emotional dimension of pain. Not only are there areas of your brain where you perceive pain but there are areas that are responsible for suffering as well. An area of your brain called the amygloid is associated with fear. Animals who have had their amygloid areas excised do not exhibit fear.

Fear, suffering and pain are in different areas of your brain but these areas are connected to each other. These interconnections ultimately can communicate with areas of your brain such as your midbrain that control your heart rate and respiratory rate as well. If you have severe pain you may sweat profusely in addition to having increases in your heart and respiratory rates. As you can see, severe pain can have adverse physiologic effects on your body. RSD/CRPS may be related to an increase in your sympathetic nervous system which may cause a profound increase in your heart rate and/or your blood pressure. These bodily changes may result in anxiety with an increase in your body's sympathetic activity. These events cause you to be in a vicious cycle. When this occurs, consultation with a psychologist is indicated.

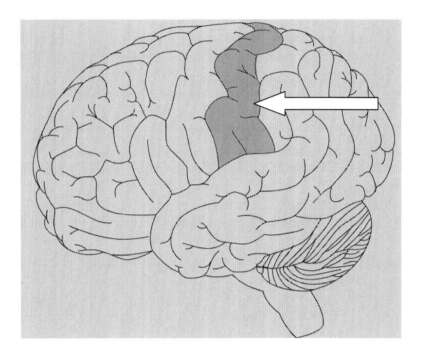

Figure 4. The brain areas (shaded) where pain signals are processed.

The transmission of pain from one part of your body to your brain is a complicated process. Remember that nerves do not touch each other. Pain signals are transmitted to your brain by chemicals that exist between your nerve endings. You can interrupt these pain signals by inhibiting the transfer of a chemical from one nerve to another. This can be done by medications, electrical stimulation, nerve blocks etc.

Pain treatment costs almost $100 billion a year in the United States. Each year, more than 500 million work days are lost, and 40 million doctor visits are made for the treatment of painful conditions. Accord-ing to the Wall Street Journal in 2001, until the past two decades no new pain treatments had been developed for more than 30 years. Since the beginning of the specialty of pain medicine, new methods for the treatment of pain have become more available. And as research is developed, new methods that have fewer side effects and are more effective are being developed. You do not need to fear a lifetime of agony as a result of your pain. Research into the processes that cause pain has resulted in the development of more drugs to block nervous system pathways that transmit pain in your body. During laboratory experiments and clinical trials, gender differences between men women are well documented with respect to pain responses. Studies of large numbers of people (epidemiological data) clearly show that women are at greater risk for developing certain pain syndromes than men and that this is believed to be a result of hormonal factors and other differences between the sexes. However, the reason why RSD/CRPS is more prevalent in women is unknown.

Pain is your body's way of telling you that something is harming your body. For example, chest pain tells you that you may be having a heart attack. Pain will cause your body to become restricted or immobile so that healing can occur. When your pain becomes severe, it tells you to seek medical attention. The problem exists when your body's pain alarm system fails to quit working and the pain continues. When pain becomes uncontrolled, depression, anxiety, and loss of sleep can result, making your perception of the pain worse. The onset of depression or anxiety happens when your pain reduces certain levels of chemicals in your brain and spinal cord. Pain is an individual experience that is difficult to study. The International Association for the Study of Pain defines pain as an unpleasant emotional and sensory experience that results from tissue injury or the threat of tissue injury.

The sensation of pain in different places on your body usually begins with the peripheral nervous system. The peripheral nervous system includes all nerves located outside of your spinal cord and brain, such as in your arms and legs. The spinal cord and brain together are called the central nervous system. Nerve fibers in the peripheral nervous system send painful impulses from nerve endings in your body directly to your spinal cord and brain.

Two main classes of nerve fibers exist that transmit pain in your body to your brain. The first class of pain fibers is called Alpha delta fibers. These fibers are able to send sharp pain and transmit pain impulses rapidly. The second class of pain fibers is called C fibers. These are smaller fibers and send burning types of pain more slowly than the Alpha delta fibers. If you were to hit your finger with a hammer, you would experience two components of pain. First, you would feel a fast, sharp pain (Alpha delta fiber), followed by a second slow, throbbing or burning (C fiber) pain. The throbbing or burning types pain last longer than sharp pain. Specific pathways exist that transmit pain information from the damaged part, or "tissue," through your spinal cord to a center of pain perception in your brain cortex called the post central gyrus. When you are hurt, chemicals called neurotransmitters are released by the injured tissue that stimulates your nerve endings to feel pain. As a result, the pain you feel comes from the place of your tissue injury. The effects of several of these neurotransmitters have been well studied. Some of these chemical substances make your nerve endings more sensitive to pain. This process is called transduction. Your body does have neurochemicals in the spinal cord that can decrease your pain intensity. Remember that pain is your body's protective mechanism to tell you that something is wrong with an area of your body. You will then protect that particular area of your body that is injured.

If a type of neurotransmitter called prostaglandin is in the painful area of your tissue, the size of your blood vessels will grow and increase your blood circulation to that area. This will cause you to have swell-ing, redness and warmth in the injured area. The pain impulse travels along the length of your nerve to a junction where the nerve enters the spinal cord. This junction between the nerve and the spinal cord is the command center for many pain syndromes. Transmission occurs when the pain impulse from the injured tissue flows to the junction at your spinal cord. From this area, the sensation of pain is transmitted to the back of your spinal cord. When the pain impulse reaches your spinal cord, it can lessen your sensation of pain. This process is called modulation.

Nerves "talk" with each another when neurotransmitter chemicals are released, causing other nerves around the injured area to transmit painful impulses. Another chemical released from injured tissue is bradykinin. Bradykinin causes C fibers to transmit pain, and also causes another type of neurotransmitter called prostaglandins to be produced. Prostaglandins decrease the level of pain tolerance that C fibers can withstand, which causes an increased sensitivity to feelings of pain. There are some medications available that can block these prostaglandins from casing pain. A common prostaglandin blocker is Ibuprofen. When the pain fibers enter the spinal cord, they terminate in different parts of the spinal cord. Ultimately these fibers will terminate in your cortex where you will experience painful sensations. Nerve cells in the spinal cord receive and respond to pain impulses from both the large and small fibers. Activation of receptors by the continual bombardment by pain impulses can result in a significant increase in your pain. The spinal cord is "upregulated" to magnify pain impulses and result in excruciating disabling pain. Dendrites carry pain toward your neuron. Axons carry pain fibers away from your neuron and direct them to the dendrites of the next neuron until they terminate in your brain or spinal cord. Remember that the axons and dendrites do not touch. They form synapses or clefts between the axon and dendrite. The synapse has chemicals in the axon nerve ending. These chemicals allow communication between the neurons. Drugs are chemicals that can interrupt the communication between the neurons at the synapses.

Another type of pain fiber exists that transmits impulses from the peripheral nervous system to the spinal cord. The third fiber that is important in understanding the transmission of pain is large nerve fibers called A beta fibers. These fibers respond to non-pain-producing stimuli such as touch, pressure or movement of joints. These fibers also end at the spinal cord. They are important because these nerves can either activate or inhibit pain impulses. The convergence of different types of nerves on your spinal cord including pain-producing nerves as well as touch and pressure producing nerves can be a source of an unusual experience referred to as referred pain.

Referred pain occurs when an individual feels pain, for example, in the shoulder when the actual pain producing tissue is the heart as is noted when an individual suffers a heart attack. This referred pain from the heart travels to the shoulder because some of the receptors in the spinal cord also receive nervous impulses from both the peripheral nervous system and arms and legs as well as within the organs within the body. In this case, the brain misinterprets the location of the injured tissue stimulus.

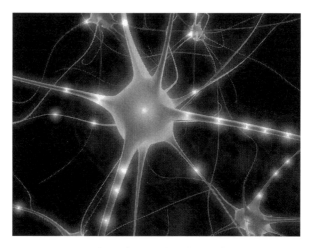

Figure 1. Neurons transmit pain and other signals throughout your nervous system. Nerves "talk" to each other by electrical signals which are generated by chemical activity.

When a hammer strikes your finger, rubbing your injured finger can result in considerable pain relief. This phenomenon was explained in 1965 by two pain researchers who published the gate-control theory of pain. Their studies revealed that only a limited amount of sensory information can be processed by the brain and spinal cord at any given moment. When pain fibers from the periphery such as the arms or legs, activate pain transmission cells in the spinal cord, signals from the non-pain-producing large fibers can inhibit or increase activation of these the pain impulses from these pain transmitting nerves. As a result, pain impulses appear to be dependent on a balance of activity in both the large and small fibers. This is the basis of the gate-control theory of pain. When the balance of nerve activity is directed toward the pain transmission fibers, the gate is open which allows transmission of painful signals to go from the spinal cord to the brain. On the other hand, when the large non-pain fibers are the dominant electrical impulses, the gate is closed and the pain signals are decreased. In some instances they may be completely blocked.

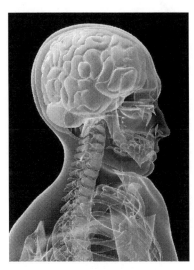

Legend for figure 2. Your central nervous system is composed of your brain and spinal cord. Pain signals travel up your spinal cord and end in your brain. Pain is perceived by your brain.

Once the pain impulses have reached your spinal cord, the pathways for pain become crossed. Pain originating from peripheral nerves on the left side of the body is transmitted to the spinal cord on the left side of the body and across the spinal cord on the right side of the body. Pain transmission then reaches the brain by two main pathways, called tracts. Chronic pain can make pain nerve endings more sensitive which results in more pain that continues to worsen over time. After a while the pain from the pain transmitting fibers can "cross wires" with the large nerves that transmit touch and movement sensation so that even a slight change in movement or light touch can cause severe agony to a patient. This is probably how RSD/CRPS patients complain of severe pain to light touch. This is called allodynia which is present in patients suffering from RSD/CRPS. Allodynia must be present for one to make a diagnosis of RSD/CRPS.

The brain and spinal cord develop when you are in your mother's womb. In other words, gender differences in body structure and brain function develop when a fetus is still in the mother's womb. These differences show themselves in childhood. These factors combine with family life-styles and school and socio-cultural sex roles to act uniquely on the individual. All of these events factor into gender-specific patterns of pain perception. During adolescence, gender differences in pain syndromes emerge, such as dysmenorrhea in women and cluster headaches in men. Smoking and other dangerous activities can influence the onset of these chronic pain syndromes in both men and women.

When acute pain becomes chronic, a self-perpetuating cycle of mala-dies can occur, resulting in changes in your body as well as behavior that make your pain worse. For example, after an injury, changes can occur in the regrowth of damaged nerve endings and where pain nerves connect with other nerves. This can result in muscle tension, making muscles extra sensitive because they are tense rather than relaxed. The increased stress from chronic pain can increase the release of a natu-rally occurring chemical in the brain called norepinepherine, eventually leading to its depletion and resulting depression and exhaustion. The depression can magnify the physical pain, which in turn depletes serotonin in both the spinal cord and brain. Persistent pain can decrease your sleep. This sleep deprivation depletes the body's supply of endorphins, which are chemicals that decrease pain. Endorphns work on pain fibers essentially like mor-phine. With the depletion of endorphins in your brain and spinal cord, your pain can become worse and you may become depressed.. As a result of the increase in pain, people often place themselves into guarded posi-tions to avoid pain. However, these unnatural positions can strain other muscles, which in turn spread more pain to other parts of the body. Other, unused muscles shrink, or atrophy, with a resulting loss of strength causing more discomfort. The goal and purpose of pain medicine is to interrupt this vicious cycle.

Endorphins, mentioned previously, can shut the gate to pain impulses. Endorphins are natural morphine like drugs (chemically related to opium) that switch off the pain alarm. Several types have been identified that modulate pain at the spinal cord and the brain. Because pain can affect breathing, blood flow, heart rate, and digestion, the body naturally re-leases endorphins to deal with pain. Moreover, pain can affect the limbic system, which is a complex area of nerve pathways in the brain that controls emotions such as mood, self preservation, rage, fear, and pleas-ure. Certain areas of the spinal cord contain high concentrations of endorphin receptors. The body also produces enkepha-lins and dynorphins, two neurochemicals also involved in pain modulation.

Another important neurochemical in RSD/CRPS pain modulation is gamma aminobutyric acid (GABA), an inhibitory pain mediator. GABA inhibits pain transmission in the spinal cord when neurons are stimulated. The nerves that conduct pain go to the spinal cord that allows pain signals to ultimately reach the brain. Areas of your body that have many pain receptors include the skin, the outer aspect of bone called the periosteum, ligaments, joints, teeth and gums and the cornea of the eye. Muscle also contains pain fibers but not as many per square meter (a measure of area) as the previously mentioned structures. Where the nerves from your body enter your spinal cord, aspartic and glutamic acid are produced. These acids increase pain impulse genera-tion. NMDA may also be produced. GABA (gamma-aminobutyric acid) in the spinal cord on the other hand, decreases the number of pain impulses that reach the brain. GABA inhibits pain impulse transmission   Norepinepherine and serotonin are two more chemicals in the spinal cord which attenuate the number of pain impulses which reach your brain. The brain and spinal cord regulate pain by the production of naturally occurring narcotic-like substances that decrease pain transmission in specific areas of the brain. These narcotic-like drugs are called enkephalins, dynorphins and beta-endorphins. Some of these substances also decrease pain transmission in the spinal cord. Enkephalins are located in areas of the brain related to pain modulation.

Enkephalins inhibit pain at the spinal cord level. Enkephalins bind to narcotic receptors. When the narcotic receptors are activated, they inhibit pain signals. Dynorphins exist in both the brain and spinal cord but are more prevalent in the brain. Like enkephalins these substances bind to narcotic receptors in the brain and spinal cord. Pain impulses that enter your spinal cord cross over to the other side and then pro-gress upward to your brain. The natural beta-endorphins in your body exhibit morphine-like activity. They work like morphine to decrease your pain. Following injury or stress these endorphins are released into the blood stream. The effects of beta-endorphins are similar to morphine. Beta-endorphins like narcotics can cause respiratory depression, constipation, euphoria, toler-ance and physical dependence. The exact biochemical actions of all of the substances mentioned are complex.

Stress can influence an animal's response to pain. There is a difference in stress-induced analgesia between male and female rodents, with the females having a greater pain response to stress. The reason for this observation is unknown and is believed not to be a result of the effect of hormones. On the other hand, estrogen, a female hormone, regulates the formation of the pain transmitter chemical substance P as well as some of the other chemicals in the nervous system that do cause pain. This may be a reason why RSD/CRPS occurs more in females than in males. Women go through a 5- to 10-year period of menopause. During this time, changes occur in hormones, most notably a decrease in the hormones in the female bloodstream. In men hormone changes occur over approximately 20 years. Body structure changes occur in both males and females. Lifestyle changes also occur during this time. Increases in the incidence of disease occur during this time in both men and women. There also is an alteration of drug metabolism in both men and women. It is interesting that the incidence of RSD/CRPS in women following menopause is the same as men.

Nicotine can have an effect on pain intensity as well in patients with RSD/CRPS. It has been shown that nicotine increases the amount of stimulus needed to cause pain in men but not in women. However nicotine can enhance a patient's sympathetic nervous system which can intensify the pain associated with RSD/CRPS.

In human patients, the over all effects of pain-relieving drugs are greater in men than in women. However, men report greater pain relief than women when morphine or morphine like drugs are used for pain control. In contrast, drugs that stimulate other receptors than the morphine receptors, such as butorphanol (Stadol), provide greater pain relief in women than men in a clinical setting. These differences in opioid medications are discussed in a later chapter. According to physiologic cardiovascular parameters in a laboratory setting, male rodents exhibit greater levels of analgesia following stressful laboratory manipulations than female rodents. This may be a result of the effects of stress on the pain systems in these animals. It is known that significant differences exist between men and women as to sensitivity to painful stimuli. Laboratory studies show that sex hormones do affect pain perception. When sex hormones are at their peak in the female, pain sensitivity is decreased.

Epidemiological studies done in 1996 and repeated in 1997 indicated that women report more severe pain intensity and more frequent pain as well as pain in multiple areas of the body and pain of a longer duration than do males. Women Reflex sympathetic dystrophy (a chronic condition that usually affects the arms or legs and causes intense aching and burning pain along with swelling, skin discoloration and temperature changes) is more prevalent in females as is a piriformis muscle syndrome (a spasm of the gluteal [buttocks] muscles). The pain stimulus differs among the sexes. Pressure and electrical pain stimuli result in larger gender-specific responses than do heat or cold stimuli. However, if heat stimuli are administered repeatedly, the gender-specific difference increases. In a laboratory setting, males demonstrate greater sensitivity than females to painful stimuli applied to areas near the genitals. A high sugar and fat intake can increase the pain in both males and females.

Phantom pain is another aspect of pain that is hard to define and note in the research lab. Phantom pain occurs after an arm, tooth or a leg is amputated. Phantom limb pain can mimic RSD/CRPS. Many patients who have had a foot amputated still complain of pain in the "foot" for many months or even years. This is due to changes within the brain and spinal cord. You may believe that the pain is in your foot even though your foot is not there, but the actual pain is experienced in areas of your brain that correspond to your foot. Right now it is not known whether women or men have a higher incidence of phantom pain. It also is not known whether hormones affect the incidence of phantom pain.

The sympathetic nervous system and its release of pain neurostimulating chemicals can increase a woman's susceptibility to reflex sympathetic dystrophy (RSD/CRPS) or causalgia as was mentioned in Chapter 1. Reflex sympathetic dystrophy and causalgia are usually caused by trauma to a nerve. These entities are more common in women. Reflex sympathetic dystrophy is a pain syndrome caused by a bruise or compression of your nerve, whereas causalgia is defined as direct trauma to your nerve (where your nerve is not completely severed). Your hormonal status at the time of a nerve injury may be important for the development of reflex sympathetic dystrophy (now called complex regional pain syndrome). Differences in the mechanisms of pain inhibition in the brain and spinal cord are presently being studied. This is important because preliminary studies have noted that equivalent doses of pain-relieving drugs differ for males and females.

The quality and intensity of pain differs for men and women which will be discussed in the next chapter.. The differences in body structure and physiology of men and women needs to be studied and further addressed, especially when developing new physical modalities as well as new drugs for the management of pain. Previous studies essentially used a majority of male subjects. No one took into consideration the differences of the effects of medications on men and women. Further studies and research into gender differences with respect to pain management may eliminate misleading information regarding the best way to manage a male's or female's pain.

It is obvious that men and women differ with respect to pain. This is also true with regard to the treatment of pain. Doctors are beginning to realize that men and women respond differently to different pain therapies. As stated earlier, the effects of the absorption and metabolism of drugs differ in men and women. It also has been mentioned that different types of drugs such as opioids and antidepressants may work differently in men and women. The menstrual cycle results in women being affected more than men with respect to the absorption of drugs through their stomach and intestine. Women experience a decreased absorption of drugs in the mid cycle of the menstrual period. When women are using hormones, there is a decreased attachment of drugs to proteins in their blood-stream after the drug has been absorbed through the intestine. Removal of drugs from the bloodstream by the kidneys appears to be equal in males and females, and this "clearance" appears to decrease as both men and women age. The treatment of RSD/CRPS may involve utilization of occupational therapy or physical therapy and sometimes chiropractor therapy. Little information is available that addresses the gender differences in the efficacy of physical therapy and chiropractic therapy. However, women are more likely to use effective forms of pain relief such as relaxation, massage, and manipulation. Studies in healthy women have demonstrated that their sensitivity to massage therapy and heat therapy can change during the menstrual cycle. Women need to consider this factor when considering the effects of heat packs or cold packs as well as massage for pain treatment.

4. Gender and Pain

Whether you are a man or a woman affects every aspect of your life. You may not realize it, but there is a difference between how and why men and women feel pain differently. For example, most women have a lower tolerance for pain than men do, but they are more sensitive and likely to express their feelings of pain than men. This means that, on average, women are more likely to recognize their long-term pain and admit to it than men. The causes and treatment of pain are different for men and women. The study of the differences between how men and women feel pain and are treated for it is a relatively new branch of medicine. Your age, physical design, hormones, psychological issues, and social issues all play a part in why you feel pain. These things also determine how your doctor will treat your pain. In the future, doctors will be able to design treatments that are specific to men and women. Simply stated, your sex (male or female) is determined by your chromosomes (XX for women, XY for men) and your body's particular anatomy. Your gender (man or woman) is determined by your body's anatomical features and social issues.

Concerning social issues, in most cases men have been programmed since they were children to be macho when dealing with pain. When playing athletic events, boys are often told to "tough it out" when they are hurt. On the other hand, women since childhood have been allowed to express their pain freely. It is socially acceptable for a girl to cry, but it is not so for a boy. These distinct differences are important when your doctor tries to figure out how to treat your pain and other medical problems. Pain is a very individual and personal experience. Things that cause pain in you may not cause pain in someone else. Without a psychological component to your type of pain, the repeated experience of the same type of pain would not be considered to be as painful as the first episode. This is the reason why a professional football player continues to play in a big game in spite of a broken bone. The psychology of the game distracts the broken-bone pain. Pain perception varies between person to person based on gender and age. When you feel pain, your response is to stay away from everything that would cause you to feel more pain. This is the response that aids your body in tissue healing. Sex differences affect the absorption, metabolism (breakdown of drugs), and excretion (elimination of drugs) of many medications. Women respond more favorably to a class of antidepressant medications called serotonin-specific reuptake inhibitors, or SSRIs (for instance, Prozac), than to other antidepressants known as tricyclics (for instance, Elavil). Sexual differences between men and women are important with respect to drug action, especially because the menstrual cycle can affect the amount of medication in the blood (blood levels).

If a female retains fluid, the excess fluid will dilute the action of the drug. Oral contraceptives (for instance, "the pill") can decrease the blood levels of some anticonvulsant medications such as Dilantin. On the other hand, oral contraceptives can increase the blood level of some medications such as Valium. Hormone replacement in women does enhance the effects of antidepressant medications. Approximately two thirds of antidepressant medications in the United States are used by women. Women have more side effects with antidepressant-type medications than men. They suffer more fatigue, gastrointestinal affects, and other adverse affects than men. Gonadal hormonal changes in women that occur monthly (before, during and after the menstrual cycle) alter the metabolism (breakdown of drugs in the liver) of certain drugs and can affect their removal from the body. One of the reasons why men and women differ in the perception of pain results from the effects of the female hormones estrogen and progesterone on the brain and spinal cord (the nervous system). The effects of the menstrual cycle on the nervous system vary before, during, and after menses. In the future, sexual and/or gender differences may allow a doctor to individualize treatments that are specific for each sex. It has also been found that low testosterone in males can also lower the pain threshold.

The wiring of the central nervous system is influenced by differences in sex. Male and female brains have approximately the same number of receptors for estrogen and androgen. Estrogen is primarily a female hormone, whereas androgen is primarily a male hormone. A receptor is an area on the outer covering, or membrane, of a cell where hormones or drugs attach and start to take action. The way receptors respond to drugs and hormones effects the body's response to both drugs and hormones. For example, giving estrogen to a man does not affect his brain like it does a woman. In the same way, giving androgens (male hormones) to a female brain does not cause the same response as in a male. Researchers have therefore concluded that hormone and hormonal receptor differences between men and women also influence the regulation and transmission of the nervous impulses that transmit pain.

Estrogen (the female hormone) affects the central nervous system levels of dopamine and serotonin, which are involved with mood disorders. Women experience more depression than males. Men may have more serotonin receptors, which may be a reason why they suffer from a lower incidence of depression. As a result, a woman's greater sensitivity to pain may be dependent on the fact that she has less serotonin in the brain and spinal cord. Studies show that sex hormones modulate neural function and affect the central nervous system with respect to the perception of pain. Recent studies in rats have shown that hormone receptors for male and female hormones are also present and modulate the function of the peripheral nerves (nerves outside the brain and spinal cord).

You are encouraged to stay informed of the new developments in gender-specific pain medicine. This will require some effort on your part. You must keep a pain diary that you can bring with you when you visit your doctor. If you have any concerns about your pain management, discuss it with your doctor. Take control of your pain by becoming better informed as to why you are suffering from pain and the methods available for the treatment of your pain. This can include not only conventional medicine, but also methods that could be offered by complementary and alternative medicine health-care providers. You should now be aware that women and men really are different. Ultimately, a better understanding of these differences will enhance your doctor's ability to diagnose and treat all types of pain. Further research should shed more light on the influence of disease on the perception of pain by men and women (and its treatment). For example, diabetes or thyroid abnormalities are diseases that ultimately can cause pain. Social issues also play a part in how pain will affect you. Pain may begin as damage to your body, but your final experience of pain will be at the brain level with your emotional feelings. Your social and cultural surroundings also can affect the emotions you have about your level of pain.

Studies into how and why men and women feel pain differently have begun in the past few years. These studies are important and must cross the life cycle of men and women, because age can also affect hormones and physical characteristics. Researchers at the University of California at

San Francisco have found that men and women respond differently to different kinds of pain-relieving medicines. Depending on the kind of medicine given, both the duration of effect and the degree to which pain was relieved differed in men and women. Pain perception will vary from person to person. While, men and women report the same number of negative (or adverse) reactions during and following treatment with therapeutic medications, negative effects of medicines are higher and more serious in women than in men. This disparity may be influenced by the fact that women use medications more often than men and in different doses, and also because the different ways the drugs are absorbed, metabolized (broken down), and removed from the body by men and women. Women often report more migraine headaches and arthritic pain than men. Women also have a greater discomfort for the same type of pain than men and are more likely to develop long-term pain after an injury. Women also use more over-the-counter pain medications and have more doctor visits than men.

Because of these differences, research (called "clinical trials" or "clinical drug research") is being done on why women are more likely to suffer from painful conditions such as RSD/CRPS than men and which medications work better for men and women. Media advertising often recommends a certain medication for a specific condition, but none of the advertisements discuss doses with respect to the body size of a man or woman. Body size determines the amount of a medicine needed to treat a painful condition. Take a look at an aspirin bottle label. Does it tell you the dosage for a man or woman? The answer is no. Reviews of major medical journals show clinical drug studies rarely test to determine how medication will affect men and women differently. Women are excluded from many clinical drug study trials. Because of the potential for pregnancy and the potential harmful effects of a new drug on a developing baby, most researchers have been hesitant to include women in their studies. Early studies mainly consisted of male prisoners.

In 1977, the U.S. Food and Drug Administration (FDA) prohibited women of child-bearing age from being involved in clinical trials. As a result, many drug studies were done only on men until recently. In 1985, a U.S. public health service task force addressed the Department of Health and Human Services and expressed the need to establish a policy that included women in clinical drug studies. In 1990, the Government Accounting

Office issued a report and concluded that there was a lack of compliance in including women in clinical drug trials. So in 1993, Congress made it mandatory that women, as well as minorities, be included in clinical drug trials. Also in 1993, the FDA began allowing women of child-bearing age to take part in clinical drug trials. In 1994, the National Institutes of Health issued guidelines to grant applications to confirm that researchers complied with the inclusion of women of child-bearing age in their studies. Recent studies in 1997 showed that women exceeded 50 percent of the study participants. (U.S. Food and Drug Administration website, www.fda.gov)

Published clinical trial results today often include data analyzing how the studied drug affected men and women. Data submitted to the FDA for drug approval must include the gender, age, height, and weight of each participant. It also has been recommended that the data include whether any participating women are pre- or postmenopausal, because levels of hormones can affect how pain much pain is felt. The anatomic differences between men and women also influence their reactions to medications. In general, women have lower body weights and organ sizes and a higher percentage of body fat, factors that need to be taken into account when discussing the way the body handles drugs and their use in men and women. For example, the muscle relaxant Valium (diazepam) causes more impairment of voluntary muscle control in women than in men, probably because of lower body weight of women as compared to men.

Differences in drug reactions are caused by differences in the way men and women process drugs. The transport of drugs within the bloodstream and the chemicals that break down drugs differ in men and women. Enzymes in the liver help break down drugs. One of these enzymes is the CYP 3A4 liver enzyme. This enzyme breaks down more than 50 percent of all therapeutic drugs. In women, drugs that have been metabolized in the liver are delivered more slowly to the bloodstream, where they are then sent to the kidneys for excretion from the body. Because more of the pain medications are not taken out of the liver, a higher concentration of these drugs in the liver requires processing. The liver enzymes in women have to process higher concentrations of the drugs than males. Liver enzymes in women may also not metabolize the antidepressants of the selective serotonin-specific reuptake inhibitor class.

Women have a lower stomach acid secretion than men. This can increase the absorption of drugs such as Elavil or Valium, and decrease the absorption of acidic drugs such as Dilantin and barbiturates. Women weigh less than men and have a lower total blood value than men. Body fat is 11 percent higher in women between the ages of 25 and 35. After a drug is absorbed from either the stomach or the small intestine, the drug is distributed throughout the tissues in the body. Drugs that have a high affinity for fat and are called fat-soluble drugs. If an individual has a high body fat content, some drugs may rapidly enter the fatty tissue. This action will decrease the level of medication in the blood and make it less effective. However, if repetitive administration of a drug causes a high concentration of that drug in body fat, it will eventually be released back into the bloodstream, which can cause a significantly higher blood level of the drug at that time.

The liver breaks down and eliminates most drugs. Biologic systems, including the liver, may be more efficient in men than in women. Drugs may be eliminated from the body more effectively by the kidneys in men when compared to women. As a result, equal doses of medication could result in a higher blood level of that particular drug in a woman than in a man. This in turn could cause serious side effects in the woman but not in the man. Alcohol is sometimes used by individuals for pain relief, too. When women smoke and consume alcohol, the effect of the tobacco enhances the effects of the alcohol, whereas in men the opposite is true. Women absorb alcohol differently than men. They also metabolize the alcohol differently than men. Women have less total body water than men at a similar body weight. Therefore, women achieve a higher concentration of the alcohol in their bloodstream after drinking an equal amount of the same alcohol. If you have less body water, the concentration of the drug in your bloodstream is higher. In other words, it is not diluted out. Males who have an increase in body water will dilute out the drug that they take. On the other hand, women eliminate alcohol from their bloodstreams faster than males.

Women experience more severe withdrawal symptoms than men when they stop smoking. Women who smoke have an increased risk of heart attack as compared to male smokers. Smoking also increases the levels of the bad cholesterol (LDL) in women more than men. Some people take illicit drugs to attempt to control their pain. Sex hormones can have an effect on illicit drugs. Women who take amphetamines say that the effects of the amphetamines differ depending on which phase of the menstrual cycle they are experiencing. Women experience fewer side effects than men when smoking cocaine. The phase of the menstrual cycle will affect whether women get high from the ingestion of cocaine. After smoking cocaine, women have a higher blood level of the drug than men. It is believed that all the effects are hormonal related.

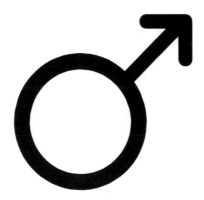

Men and women differ with respect to their response to medications. Note, therefore, that the dosage for men and women must differ. However, many doctors are unaware of the gender-specific differences between men and women with respect to their responses to medications, as well as the differences between men and women with respect to body weight. An obese woman may require more medication to achieve the same pain relief than a thin woman. Before men and women with painful conditions can be treated properly, many research questions need to be answered with respect to the different effects of drugs on men and women. As you can see, attention to gender is important not only in the specialty of pain management but also in other medical specialties. Sex hormones influence the effects of analgesics and many other drugs. The menstrual cycle, pregnancy, and menopause affect how drugs react in women's bodies, such that the same drug will have a different effect depending on the stage of the menstrual cycle and whether the woman is pre- or postmenopausal. When you take a pill, the amount of medication that you are taking may not be appropriate for you depending on the previously mentioned factors. This may be the reason why a drug "just stops working." In some instances, if you mention this to your doctor, the doctor may think you are just seeking more drugs. The way in which antidepressant medications are absorbed, distributed in the bloodstream, and eliminated by the kidneys differs in men and women. Monthly hormone cycles in women can influence the effects of some antidepressants. Further, oral contraceptives and hormones can alter drug interactions in women. For example, acetaminophen (Tylenol) is made inactive in women taking oral contraceptives when compared to women who are not taking oral contraceptives. High blood levels of estradiol (a female hormone) sensitize a female to thermal (heat) pain.

Premenopausal women take longer to empty stomach content such as food and medication. In essence, this means that medications in the stomach are slower to leave the stomach to go into the small intestine. The small intestine has a greater absorptive capacity than the stomach. If a medication is delayed in passage from the stomach to the small intestine, medicine will be absorbed more slowly into the blood. Consequently, the blood level of the drug may be decreased. The effects of hormones on neurotransmitters in the brain during the premenstrual cycle can affect the sensitivity of neurotransmitters or nervous system receptors. A doctor may have to increase the total dosage of a specific medication throughout the entire menstrual cycle and may have to decrease the medication two to three days after the cycle has been completed. Oral contraceptives used by some women can decrease the effect of anti-anxiety drugs such as the Valium. Studies are currently investigating whether estrogen can be effective in treating depression in women. The effects of estrogen on certain drugs in postmenopausal women is also currently under study. Men and women respond differently to antidepressant medications. In women, pre- and post-menopausal effects must be taken into account when prescribing an antidepressant medication.

Age also influences the effects of drugs. Because older people break down drugs more slowly, older individuals typically need a smaller dose of a drug. However, age effects are less prevalent in women than in men. Older men have a decreased ability to excrete drugs than women. Age can also influence how sensitive you may be to pain. The intensity of pain felt by children lessens as they grow older. As puberty approaches, girls will notice and report more pain than boys do. Osteoarthritis, which affects 40 percent of middle-age patients and approximately 70 percent of geriatric patients, essentially will have the same degree of input into the central nervous system of men and women. However, patient responses to the degree of pain differs. Women appear to cope better with pain related to osteoarthritis than men.

A study in Sweden published in 2002 reported that gender bias can occur in a doctor's management of pain. In the study, men and women were treated differently by some doctors because of a gender-stereotyped attitude. Both men and women doctors contributed to the gender-disparate treatment. According to this study, male doctors emphasize the importance of patient compliance to female patients, whereas female doctors emphasize the importance of patient compliance to male patients. The investigators involved in the study concluded that gender differences should be taught in medical school to promote awareness of this problem.

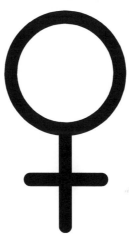

Pain medicine is in its infancy, as is gender-specific medicine. Treatment methods are constantly changing. It is unknown why females have a higher incidence of RSD/CRPS than males. Do as much research as you can to learn about the different methods available for you to treat your RSD/CRPS pain. Feel free to discuss them with your doctor and ask any questions that you may have. Understanding your condition will help you to take charge of your own treatment and help make that treatment as successful as possible.

You should realize that your pain management should be tailored to your age, gender psychological makeup etc. The "one size fits all" mentality of some physicians is not acceptable in modern medicine.

5. Pain Assessment

Most pain assessments are done in the form of a scale. The scale is explained to the patient and they give a score. A rating is taken before administering any medication and after the specified time frame to rate the efficacy of a treatment. RSD/CRPS can be very painful. Several different techniques are available for your doctor to use in determining your level of pain. Commonly used techniques include verbal, visual, and psychological tests. Both you and your doctor are responsible for documenting and recording trends in the intensity and frequency of your pain. This information tells each of you whether your pain has really improved or whether it has worsened. Charting your pain levels will help your doctor see your long-range pain trends, which are ultimately more important than your day-to-day pain trends.

You may wonder why you need to measure your pain. A pain-experience measurement is extremely valuable to both you and your doctor. It provides a baseline for your doctor to assess any therapy or medications you are currently taking, and it also helps your doctor to prescribe future therapy methods. Your doctor also needs to be able to determine how much disability you have in order to prescribe the appropriate types of therapy for you. Many of the test instruments that mentioned in this chapter enable doctors to diagnose a specific pain condition. They also help doctors determine whether the patient is truly in pain or just making it up. You should be able to easily understand the test you are being given so that it is as accurate as possible at measuring your level of pain.

After reading this chapter you will be able to see that you and your doctor can use several different pain-assessment forms to monitor your pain-medicine therapy. Which form is best for you? There is no definite answer to this question. The assessment form that you feel most comfortable with and one that you will use is the best pain assessment for both you and your doctor. These assessment scales help you and your doctor plan an individualized pain-management program. Look over your pain-assessment evaluations carefully. If you are not decreasing your pain, or if your pain is becoming worse, you and your physician must evaluate other treatments for your pain. You and your doctor must develop a partnership in the control of your pain.

Your doctor will depend on you for accurate and reliable answers to questions about the pain you feel. Because pain involves many aspects such as sensory, emotional, and behavioral factors, it is difficult to measure the amount of pain you feel based on one thing. Your doctor will carefully instruct you as to how to report your pain when going through a pain-assessment test. The choice of a pain-assessment test depends on the needs of both you and your doctor. Two common tests are a Number Scale and a Faces Scale. Using a Number Scale, patients rate pain on a scale from 0-10, 0 being no pain and 10 being the worst pain ever imaginable. The Faces Scale is a scale with corresponding faces depicting various levels of pain is shown to the patient and they select one.

A functional evaluation, such as reports of your daily activities, must be included in your assessment. If your doctor does not ask about your daily activities, voluntarily tell him your further limitations with respect to work, recreation, dressing, fixing meals, and any other daily activities. Use a daily pain diary and tell your doctor whether your pain is becoming worse or is getting better. This will enable your doctor to assess your medication and therapy needs. Positive effects of therapy are best assessed when your doctor keeps a database of your pain progression. This type of data is easily stored on a computer. This type of database is even more valuable because your doctor can graph important data from each of your visits.

The assessment and measurement of pain has received considerable attention in the past two decades. Progress continues to be made in developing pain-assessment tools. You or your doctor should not over-simplify your pain assessment. The objective reports you are able to give, as well the observations your doctor is able to make about your behavior, are important to accurate pain management decisions. Because pain is subjective and can be observed only by you, it is important that the reports of your pain levels come from you. This will give your doctor a more accurate measurement of the type of pain you are experiencing. For example, if you just complain of a toothache, your doctor will have almost no way of knowing how severe your pain is. On occasion, your doctor will need to rate your level of pain if you are not able for some reason to identify your level of pain. In general, you should be able to accurately describe your level of pain. If you are not able to rate your pain yourself, it should be done only by your doctor or other type of health-care provider. Each doctor's approach to managing pain may differ. Therefore, it is important that you and your doctor have a healthy doctor-patient relationship and that your doctor understands your situation. The situations and causes of each person's pain differ, and therefore your doctor may suggest different combinations of methods to help relieve your pain.

The current methods doctors have available to measure your pain are imperfect. The perception of pain is based on many things that affect you, and can range from memories of a previous painful event to psychological influences. Pain is not necessarily just a sensory experience, but it is also a result of processes that occur at a higher level in the brain, making pain a psychological experience. There is no general consensus among pain medicine doctors as to the best test for the measurement of pain. An ideal test for the assessment of pain must bring together experimental as well as clinical knowledge. Right now, there are no adequate tests that can differentiate gender with respect to the assessment of pain. In order to provide adequate pain management, a doctor must combine all of the data given by you concerning your pain complaints.

Hopefully a universally accepted pain assessment test will become available in the near future. In the meantime, you and your doctor must talk not only about pain complaints, but also about your feelings of depression and anxiety during each office visit. You and your doctor must develop a healthy relationship so that the appropriate pain modalities can be rationally prescribed specifically for you. Pain is subjective and does not allow itself to be measured accurately. In other words, it is impossible to visualize "pain." When your doctor interviews you about your pain complaints, he or she will begin by asking the following questions: the time of the onset of your pain, the location of the pain on your body, how long it lasts, and how often it occurs during the day.

Your doctor also will ask you whether your pain is sharp, dull, or cramping. You should tell your doctor whether your pain is mild, moderate, or severe. Women in general are more able to express their pain experiences than men. You must provide your doctor with enough information so that he or she can come up with a reasonable and accurate diagnosis for you.

What follows is an initial pain-assessment form. This assessment addresses your pain and psychosocial issues and leaves room for your doctor's evaluation of your condition. Your doctor will give you a copy of this assessment form. You will be asked questions such as when the pain began, how long it lasts, what makes it worse, what makes it better, what medications you are taking, what effects medications are having on your pain, and what your emotional status is during episodes of pain.

One way of assessing your pain is to use a numeric scale. This is the simplest method for attempting to measure your pain. During this test, you are asked to rate your pain on a scale of 0 to 5 or to use words such as "none," "slight," "moderate," or "severe." This assessment is also a quick, simple, and reliable way to evaluate the effectiveness of any medications you are taking to manage your pain. On the numeric scale, 0 equals no pain, 1 equals mild pain, 2 equals moderate pain, 3 equals distressing pain, 4 equals horrible pain, and 5 equals excruciating pain confining you to bed rest. This method is easily understood and may be helpful in guiding the treatment plans your doctor creates for you. Another type of verbal scale asks you to rate your pain on a scale of 1 to 10, with 1 being equivalent to pain that is barely noticeable, and 10 relating to excruciating pain. A verbal numeric scale is easily understood. All you have to do is choose a number to represent your level of pain.

The following numeric pain intensity scale is the most popular test used by pain-medicine specialists. You circle a number on the scale that corresponds to how much pain you feel. It only uses numbers from 0 through 10 along the length of the horizontal scale. A score of 0 indicates no pain, whereas a score of 10 means that you feel the worst pain ever imagined. Another method used by some doctors is a pain diary. This is a descriptive report you keep to assess your pain. The pain diary shows a written account of your day-to-day experiences. It can be used to help diagnose the cause of your pain. The value of the pain diary is that you and your doctor can monitor your day-to-day variation of painful states and your response to therapy. You need to keep a diary of your pain patterns when you are sitting, standing, and lying down. Also record sleep patterns and sexual activity. You also must note the amount of pain medication you are taking and whether it lessens your pain. Because pain can interfere with eating patterns, keep a diary of the amount of food you eat and at what time you ate. Be sure to include any types of recreational activities and whether your pain felt better or worse afterward. You have to be diligent in your record keeping. This form enables you to record an entire month of pain-intensity scores, your activities, the location of your pain, and a medication log. Your physician will find this diary extremely helpful in working with you to plan your pain therapy.

Pain drawings offer a visual way to evaluate your pain. You will be asked to shade in areas on a human figure outline that correspond to the areas of your pain. The drawing will help your doctor determine where your pain is coming from and how widespread it is on your body. Over time, your pain drawings can be compared to show the changes of your pain and how you are responding to therapy. The following is a sample pain-assessment tool that includes diagrams for you to shade to tell your doctor whether your pain is confined to one area of your body or whether your pain is widespread throughout your body. This form allows you to shade the areas of your body where you are feeling your pain. A common method of determining the behavioral component of your pain is for you to be directly observed by your doctor. You must be observed while sitting, walking to and from the office, and getting in and out of vehicles. Your doctor will focus his or her attention on the area of your major pain complaint.

Behavioral influences affecting your perception of pain include the amount of medications you use and the number of doctor visits required. Limping and facial grimacing also are appropriate behavioral evaluations of pain. Depression and anxiety are emotional factors that can be measured by tests. Because the experience of pain is impossible to measure directly, your doctor must observe your displays of appropriate or inappropriate physical behavior. After observing your behavior, your doctor may classify you using the following four-class system: Class 1 consists of patients with low physical injury but high levels of abnormal behavior patterns related to their pain. Class 2 consists of patients with lower physical injury and low behavior pattern abnormalities. Class 3 consists of patients with significant tissue injury in addition to high behavioral pattern abnormalities. Class 4 consists of patients with a high tissue injury and a normal behavioral patterns.

A visual analog scale is another method of assessment that attempts to measure your level of pain. Instead of choosing a number, you are asked to mark a point on a horizontal line that is labeled with "no pain" at one end and "the worst possible pain" at the opposite end. The line is divided into 10 equal spaces, and you choose number from 1 to 10 based on your level of pain. It is slightly more difficult to administer than the numeric method, but some doctors and researchers think that the visual analog scale is more accurate than the numeric scale for pain measurements. On the following form you will circle a point on the line that indicates how much pain you feel. Descriptive words are placed along the horizontal scale, which enables you to describe the severity of your pain. Another visual scale that is easy to use, especially for children, is the face scale. It shows pictures of happy to grimacing faces and patients are asked to circle the face that shows what kind of pain they feel. Using descriptive words is one method of describing your pain. Self-reports have been used by doctors since 1939. A pain-rating index consists of groups of words associated with pain. This index has been incorporated into the McGill pain questionnaire, a type of verbal assessment that uses word descriptors that are valuable in discriminating between different pain syndromes. For the following pain assessment form you will circle the words that best describe your pain. Since they are in no particular order, there is no obvious progression of pain shown.

A McGill pain questionnaire is a method for assessing pain psychologi-cally. A McGill pain questionnaire gives a multidimensional pain score. You are given 20 word sets that describe a different dimension of your pain. You are asked to select words relevant to your pain from each of these 20 sets. For example, one set includes the words "jumping," "flash-ing," and "shooting." Another set includes the words "tingling," "itching," "smarting," and "stinging." You circle the word that relates closest to the pain you feel throughout the 20 word sets. This questionnaire is difficult to administer as well as to interpret. However, it has characteristic re-sponse patterns for different pain syndromes such as back pain, arthritis, and cancer. The validity of this questionnaire continues to be studied. The McGill pain questionnaire consists of four different parts. The first part consists of a human figure drawing on which you are instructed to mark the location of your pain. The second part is the pain-rating index that contains 78 words divided into 20 groups. Each set contains up to six words. Five of these groups describe tension or fear. Each word is as-signed a value according to its position within a subclass. The third part of this test asks additional questions about prior pain experiences, as well as the location of the pain and current usage of pain medications. The fourth part consists of a present pain intensity index. This aspect of the test requests a pain score from 0 to 5 with word descriptors such as no pain, mild pain, discomforting pain, distressing pain, or horrible and excruciating pain. These words also are assigned different values. All the values are added to obtain a total score. All the scores are then evaluated to attempt to assess your total pain experience. The problem with this test is that there is no specific mechanism within the test itself to determine which component truly reflects your pain experience. The value of this test, however, is that it treats pain as a multidimensional experience. There also is a short form of the McGill pain questionnaire that has been developed. This questionnaire contains fewer words and categories than the long form. This test is sensitive to evaluations of reduction in pain experiences. This test is more useful for rapid evaluation of data following procedures or surgery.

Some simple tests have been developed that your physician can administer in his or her office. These test are not as comprehensive as the McGill Questionnaire but do give a quick estimate of how your pain compares with other pain patients. Certain psychological tests exist , including the P-3® and the BBHITM that assist healthcare practitioners in the assessment of biopsychosocial factors that can affect the effective diagnosis and treatment of your pain.   You must realize that if your physician requires you to take a psychological test that he or she does not think that you are imagining your pain. The goal is to determine how much suffering you are experiencing as a result of your pain syndrome. This information is helpful in planning an overall treatment plan for you.

The following is a pain diary that may be of some help to you and your physician. You should fill the form out daily; when you awaken, at noon and in the evening. You are instructed to rate your pain on a score from 0 to 10 with 0 being no pain and 10 the worst imaginable. You can create your own pain diary using a computer spreadsheet program or a word processing program. Some patients like to use a notebook. Some patients prefer to graph their pain scores to watch their pain trends. No matter which pain diary that you use, you need some data to give to your physician, therapist and/or chiropractor so that any further treatment can be assessed. You can create your own pain diary as below. Go to The AGS Foundation for Health in Aging at www.healthinaging.org

Daily Pain Assessment

Date_____

Time	Where is the pain? Rate the pain (0- 10), or list the word from the scale that describes your pain.	What were you doing when the pain started or increased?	Did you take medicine? What did you take? How much?	What other treatments did you use?	After an hour, what is your pain rating?	Other problems or side effects? Comments.
Morning						
Noon						
Evening						

6.   Causes of RSD/CRPS

Reflex sympathetic dystrophy is a form of neuropathic pain in which the pain and hyperalgesia experienced by a patient are dependent on sympathetic innervation of the painful area. Sprouting of sympathetic fibers serves as a coupling link between the sympathetic system and the sensory system and is believed to be an important neurological mechanism underlying reflex sympathetic dystrophy. Although inflammatory cytokines play a pivotal role in the initiation of sympathetic sprouting, the underlying mechanisms are not clear. Evidence suggests that cyclo-oxygenases especially cytokines-inducible COX-2, are causal factors that contribute to the development of neuropathic pain. COX2 can be expressed in the lumbar ganglia resulting from the synthesis and release of inflammatory cytokines following peripheral nerve injury. Up-regulated expression of COX-2 will induce the sprouting of the sympathetic efferent axons and leads to pain.

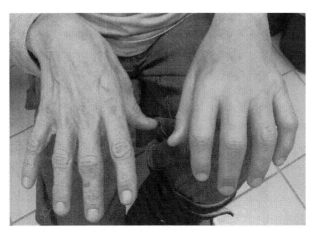

Figure 1. The left hand demonstrates an early stage of RSD/CRPS. This individual fell when he tripped over a bicycle lying in his driveway.

Reflex sympathetic dystrophy and causalgia were originally described by Dr. Mitchell, a neurologist during the Civil War. He noted that some soldiers who had injuries to their hands or feet developed a syndrome that consisted of burning pain, pain to touch over the skin of the injured extremity, shiny skin, and skin that had different colors consisting of either redness or a blue cyanotic color. Dr. Mitchell also noted that the pain in the extremity was out of proportion to the injury. For example, if you sustained a sprain to your ankle, you would expect to have some pain. However, if you develop reflex sympathetic dystrophy, the pain is excruciating and unbearable. The pain is out of proportion to your injury.

Reflex sympathetic dystrophy (RSD) can be a devastating entity for you, especially if it is not diagnosed and treated within a timely fashion. Reflex sympathetic dystrophy usually affects one of your extremities (arms or legs) but also can affect your face as well. Reflex sympathetic dystrophy is now called complex regional pain syndrome (CRPS). RSD/CRPS is a chronic, painful, and progressive neurological condition that affects skin, muscles, joints, and bones. Pain associated with this entity is throbbing, burning, or aching. You can have pain just to light touch. This is termed allodynia. You can have swelling of your extremity as well as either warmth or coldness depending on the phase of your RSD/CRPS and sweating. Your hair may grow faster on the extremity with RSD/CRPS at first, only to slow down as the disease progresses. Your extremity will sweat which is termed hyperhidrosis. It can turn a reddish or blue (cyanotic) color. The nails in your affected limb can grow faster on the extremity that suffers from reflex sympathetic dystrophy. The syndrome usually develops in an injured limb, such as a broken leg, or following surgery. However, many cases of RSD involve only a minor injury, such as a sprain. And in some cases, no precipitating event can be identified. The International Association for the Study of Pain clinical criteria for RSD/CRPS is as follows: the presence of regional pain and sensory changes following a noxious event, pain is associated with associated findings such as abnormal skin color, temperature change, abnormal sudomotor activity, edema, no distribution of the pain of a single nerve in the extremity and the combination of these findings exceeds their expected magnitude in response to known physical damage during and following the inciting event. Pain may begin in one area or limb and then spread to other limbs. RSD/CRPS is characterized by various degrees of burning pain, excessive sweating, swelling, and sensitivity to touch. Symptoms of RSD/CRPS may recede for years and then reappear with a new injury. RSD/CRPS is potentially disabling. Two types of RSD/CRPS have been defined: Type 1; is RSD/CRPS without nerve injury and Type 2 (causalgia) is RSD/CRPS with a nerve injury. Reflex sympathetic dystrophy usually occurs following an injury. However, a heart attack or stroke can cause you to have reflex sympathetic dystrophy.

It can be seen in the knee as well as in the shoulder. In a study of reflex sympathetic dystrophy, 40 percent of the cases followed an injury to a muscle or a nerve. Simple bruises or sprains can trigger reflex sympathetic dystrophy. Fractures accounted for 25 percent of reflex sympathetic dystrophy cases.

Twenty percent of RSD/CRPS patients are postoperative on an arm or leg, whereas 12 percent occurred after a heart attack. Three percent occurred after a stroke. RSD/CRPS affects both men and women, and also occurs in children. It can occur at any age, but usually affects people between the ages of 40 and 60 years and is more prevalent in females. The National Institute of Neurological Disorders and Strokes (NINDS) reports that 2% to 5% of peripheral nerve injury patients and 12% to 21% of patients with paralysis on one side of the body (hemiplegia) develop reflex sympathetic dystrophy as a complication. The Reflex Sympathetic Dystrophy Syndrome Association of America (RSDSA) reports that the condition appears after 1% to 2% of bone fractures. As you can see the injury that precedes the onset of RSD/CRPS may or may not be significant. It was once thought that reflex sympathetic dystrophy was an emotional problem. However, studies have shown that many people do not suffer from emotional problems at the time of onset of reflex sympathetic dystrophy. To prevent you from having permanent disability, treatment needs to be started immediately. RSD/CRPS appears to involve the complex interaction of the sensory, motor, and autonomic nervous systems, and the immune system. It is thought that brain and spinal cord (central nervous system) control over these various processes is somehow changed as a result of an injury. It was originally hypothesized that if your sympathetic nervous system became hyperactive, this hyperactivity was at least one of the causes of reflex sympathetic dystrophy. Your sympathetic nervous system is one component of your autonomic nervous system. The other component of your autonomic nervous system is called the parasympathetic nervous system. Your autonomic nervous system regulates your circulation and your breathing as well as your stomach and bladder functions. You have no control over your autonomic nervous system. This distinguishes it from your peripheral nervous system that is usually under your control.

The symptoms of RSD/CRPS may progress through three stages; acute, dystrophic, and atrophic. The acute stage occurs during the first 1-3 months and is a hyperdynamic state. An increased blood flow to the affected anatomic site is noted. You may have burning pain, swelling, increased sensitivity to touch, increased hair and nail growth in the affected region, joint pain, and color and temperature changes. A triple phase bone scan or laser Doppler imaging study will demonstrate blood flow. The dystrophic stage may involve constant pain and swelling. The onset of this stage is 3-6 months following the onset of the original symptoms. The affected anatomic part usually feels cool to touch and looks cyanotic. You may experience muscle stiffness and wasting as well as osteoporosis. During the atrophic stage which usually occurs after six months, the skin becomes cool and shiny, increased muscle stiffness and weakness occur, and the symptoms may spread to another limb or limbs.

The diagnosis of RSD/CRPS is by clinical examination. There is no single test that will make the diagnosis. Physical examination involves observing the skin color and temperature, swelling, and vascular reactivity, overgrown and grooved nails; swollen and stiff joints, muscle weakness and atrophy and muscle spasms. A MRI scan may demonstrate bone marrow edema. Thermography may be helpful as is laser Doppler Imaging for evaluating RSD/CRPS. The goals of treatment are to control pain and to maintain as much mobilization of the affected limb as possible. An individualized treatment plan is designed, which often combines physical therapy, medications, nerve blocks, and psychosocial support. In 1916, a surgeon described that reflex sympathetic dystrophy pain could be relieved by surgically removing some of the sympathetic fibers that innervate the affected extremity. This surgeon also noted that patients who had this procedure had some pain relief and had decreased sweating and improvement in their skin color. This surgeon then thought that the sympathetic nervous system was involved in the etiology of reflex sympathetic dystrophy.

In 1995, another doctor described another method using a scope for the removal of sympathetic nerve fibers that innervate your limb that has RSD/CRPS, and this has became a standard treatment for reflex sympathetic dystrophy. Over time the treatment of reflex sympathetic dystrophy included repet-tive sympathetic blocks such as stellate ganglion blocks or removal of the sympathetic nerves, either surgically or by chemicals such as phenol. These procedures for many years have been the standard treatment for the treatment of reflex sympathetic dystrophy. Finally, doctors who regularly treat reflex sympathetic dystrophy critically evaluated the effectiveness of these procedures. It is now known that temporary relief can occur with these procedures, but long-term results are poor. It is possible that these procedures have only survived time as a standard treatment for RSD because of the lack of more effective therapy. Furthermore, for years research on reflex sympathetic dystrophy was lacking because it was thought that this entity was mainly of a psychological origin. For sympathetic blockade to be effective, blockade must be done soon after the diagnosis of RSD/CRPS. After 12-16 weeks blockade becomes ineffective. Some patients can have sympathetic independent pain. In these instances sympathetic blockade has no effect. This does not mean that a patient does not have RSD/CRPS is they have no response to blockade. It only means that the patient has a version of RSD/CRPS called sympathetic independent pain. Therefore, there is no reason for a physician to keep doing multiple injections.

COX-2 inhibitors such as Celebrex (celecoxib) and an anticonvulsant like gabapentin can be effective for pain contro. Insomina can be managed with tricyclic medications. Nonin-flammatory pain can be treated with tramadol. Steroids can be effective in the acute stage of RSD/CRPS. Steroids can keep inflammatory cytokines from being produced. Muscle cramps can be treated with baclofen. Medications that affect the sympathetic nervous system such as clonidine in the form of a transdermal patch can be useful in some cases. Each of these drugs may be medically necessary. Physical therapy and/or occupational therapy should be used to mobilize the affected part and preserve range of motion.

Pain that is out of control following an injury to an upper or lower extremity should alert a physician, a patient, a case worker and/or adjuster that RSD/CRPS may be beginning. At that time the injured person must be referred to a health care provider knowledgeable in the diagnosis and treatment of RSD/CRPS. The prognosis with early treatment is excellent if treatment is initiated in a timely fashion. Otherwise, These cases can be very expen-sive requiring dorsal column stimulator placement and life long therapies and medications. A surgical sympathectomy has not been shown to provide long term relief.

A transcutaneous electrical nerve stimulation (TENS) unit may be used to treat the affected area. Severe pain can cause depression as well.

RSD/RSD patients often become depressed and anxious because of chronic pain and loss of physical ability. Counseling, support groups, and chronic pain center programs help patients learn coping strategies and provide emotional and psychological support. You need to be aware that spontaneous remission can occur after several weeks to months. There is usually no question that a work related injury can cause the RSD/CRPS. An explanation of causation is presented subsequently. You will see how difficult it is to assign causation. Why does a small percentage of the population with similar fractures develop RSD/CRPS? If you suspect RSD/CRPS you must act accordingly as in many instances, the treating physician fails to make the diagnosis. If a prompt and accurate diagnosis is not made the financial liability of the insurance company may devastating. Robert, a 55 year old male has increasing hand pain, redness and swelling. He has a fracture of his left wrist. His uncle has a history of RSD/CRPS. He smokes two packs of cigarettes per day. He fell at the place of his employment while he was on his lunch hour. Who should assume the financial liability for his newly reported medical condition? What caused his RSD/CRPS? Knowledge of causation is important. This chapter is concerned with medical causation. However, you need to have some knowledge of legal causation. Legal causation is not medical causation.

The understanding of causation is important in understanding the causes of injuries or diseases in individuals. However, you need to understand causation as it applies to groups in the population as well. In this case you need to understand a model of causation. If you can help define the causative factor leading to injury in a certain population of individuals then by discussing the problem with the employer, maybe the injuries can be prevented. Such as the fall just mentioned This is what preventive medicine specialists do. The determination of causation is difficult to determine in general. The diagnosis of RSD/CRPS is difficult because it is a rare entity. You need to know what event caused the individual's medical condition in order for you to establish causation. For example, the multi-factorial nature of low back pain and our ignorance with the spectrum of contributing factors to the low back pain makes it difficult to specify the exact cause of a specific condition. The same is true with RSD/CRPS causation.

You can use the "but for" theory in the case example presented (a result would not have happened but for the occurrence of a certain event). Is the cause of the workers' low back pain related to the occurrence of occasionally lifting 40 pound boxes? If they never lifted heavy boxes, would they have low back pain? Did the fall cause the RSD/CRPS? People fall frequently, but only a few develop RSD/CRPS. The addition of multiple similar claims in the same work environment makes the determination of causation more difficult. Causation is an event that produces an effect. In other words causation is an event that causes something to happen. Determination of causation is straightforward in some cases and not so with others. Decisions regarding opinions for causation are based on "reasonable medical certainty" and when possible through evidence based literature or scientific research. You need to be aware that some conditions may be related to one's occupation but may also occur within a normal population. Up to 85% of individuals who report back pain, no pain-producing pathology can be identified; conversely, some 30% of asymptomatic people have significant pathology on imaging studies scans that might be expected to cause back pain. Causal relevance helps explain if and why one event caused another event. If you want to know why an airplane crashed for example, you will seek an antecedent event that could have caused the accident such as inclement weather, ice on the wings or runway, engine malfunction etc.

Causation implies that a set of circumstances exist that in their presence a specific effect occurs and in their absence, the effect does not occur. Remember that RSD/CRPS can occur with no injury. A litmus paper in a chemistry lab always turns a specific color when placed in an acidic or basic solution. The solution always causes a specific effect when it comes in contact with litmus paper. Otherwise, a change in the color of the litmus paper does not occur. Plain water will not change the litmus paper color. The acidic solution causes the litmus paper to turn red. A cause does not have to come before an effect as they can both occur at the same time. You need to know the difference between a necessary cause and a sufficient cause. A factor may be a sufficient cause or a necessary cause to produce an effect. If two or more conditions is necessary for a given effect, no one condition on its own causes the effect.

A necessary condition is a single specific condition that is necessary for an effect to occur. An example is treatment of a lethal disease. The disease cannot be cured without drug A. Therefore, drug A is a necessary medicine to cause a cure of the disease. If one or more drugs together can cure the disease and no one drug on its own cures the disease then the drugs as a group are necessary to cure the disease but each drug is sufficient to affect the disease. If a condition occurs, then the effect must occur with respect to the list of drugs. Each is sufficient to cure the diseases. An effect may have a multitude of sufficient causes. A metal wire is necessary to conduct electricity but silver, lead and aluminum are all themselves sufficient to conduct electricity. You should try and know all of the conditions possible to give a specified effect in a case that you may be involved with. If a claimant has degenerative disc disease you should be aware of all the etiologies of degenerative disc disease.

Mill in 1843 presented four methods to show causation.

1.   Method of agreement: A certain factor is necessary for a certain effect and the factor in question is always present when the effect is present.

2.   Method of difference: The factor present when the effect occurs is always absent when the effect is absent.

3.   Method of agreement and difference: The factor causing the effect is always present when the effect is present and is always absent when the effect is absent.

4.   Method of concomitant variation: A certain factor necessary to cause a certain effect varies in a direct relationship with the degree of effect.

All relevant factors that can cause an event must be correctly identified before determining which event if any caused the result. You must analyze the resultant effect using a set of causal factors.

You furthermore, need to understand the difference between causation and correlation. A correlation exists between smoking and lung cancer. Correlation is based on percentages. A high percentage of people for example, who smoke, develop lung cancer. However, all smokers do not develop lung cancer and people who develop lung cancer do not have to have a smoking history to develop lung cancer. Therefore, the act of smoking does not always cause lung cancer but a positive correlation exists between smoking and lung cancer. The argument for causation is : If event A then event B. The argument for correlation is: If event A than probably event B. Figures 1 and 2 will present graphically, these differences.

You need to be aware of two possible errors in establishing causation. Causal fallacies require your attention and need to be recognized. The first error is post hoc fallacy which means "after this, therefore because of this". It is a fallacy to conclude that because one event happened after another event occurred before the second event that the first event caused the second event. An example is having an accident after a black cat crosses your path. The cat did not cause your accident and it is a fallacy to think that it did. The second error is that it is a also a fallacy to confuse a cause with a correlation. A correlation does not necessarily imply a cause. A correlation is a mutual relation. An example is that from 1840 until 1963 every president elected in a year ending in 0 died in office. President Regan was subsequently elected in a year that did end in 0 and did not die in office. Therefore, being elected in a year ending in 0 does not cause one to die while in office but a correlation exists nevertheless.

Causation must be specific enough to distinguish causation from mere correlation. Correlation is a simultaneous change in the value of two random variables and is described as positive or negative. An example of a positive correlation is the relationship between cigarette smoking and lung cancer. As the incidence of smoking increases, the incidence of lung cancer increases. A negative correlation example is the correlation between age and normal vision. As a patient ages, vision decreases in a certain percentage of patients. Correlation involves a mutual or common relationship. Causation on the other hand does not. Causation is an essential concept in epidemiology (a science that studies the causes of disease, death etc), yet there is no single, clearly articulated definition for the discipline. From a systematic review of the literature, five categories of causation can be described: probabilistic, counterfactual dependence, instrumental, singularist and insufficient but non redundant.

Probabilistic causation is one type of causation and describes causality as a probable occurrence. The basic idea of the probabilistic approaches to causation is that a cause is an event A, the occurrence of which makes the occurrence of event, B, more likely than if A had not occurred. Because probability necessarily implies a range of events, this view is usually expressed in terms of types of events. Smoking for example can cause lung cancer. Probablistic causation implies therefore that the probability of getting lung cancer is higher for those who smoke than for those who do not. As a result, one event may be said to be a cause of another event if, given the occurrence of the first event, the probability of the occurrence of the resultant event is higher than the probability of the occurrence of the second event would have occurred if the initial event had not occurred. The probabilistic definition is consistent with scientific and public health goals of epidemiology. In debates in the literature over these goals, proponents of epidemiology as a pure science favor a probabilistic method.

Another type of causality is counterfactual dependence. To say that a resultant event is causally dependent upon a prior event is to say that if a prior event had not occurred, then the resultant event would not have occurred. Moreover, to say that the antecedent event is the cause of the resultant event is to state that there is a chain of causally dependent events linking the initial event with the final event. For example, an injured worker has a herniated lumbar disc noted on his MRI. He sustained a lifting injury with a history of a "pop" in his back and the sudden onset of pain in the back of his leg immediately after lifting a heavy box at work. The disc herniation was caused by a prior event (the act of lifting).

Cause can be insufficient but non redundant. If a fire marshal declares that a short-circuit was the cause of a fire, this individual says that the short-circuit is a condition that occurred and that other conditions which also form a sufficient condition for a fire such as oxygen, combustible materials etc. were also present, and that no other sufficient condition of the house's catching fire was present at the time that the fire occurred.

The instrumental approach is another type of causality. The main point of this approach is that there are causes only for persons who are concerned with certain kinds of events. Consequently, what may be the cause of an event in the eyes of one person, may not be the cause from the point of view of another. For example a worker with a history of severe degenerative disc disease who develops back pain while sitting at his work station.

The worker assumes that the cause of his back pain is work related. On the other hand his case worker and adjuster conclude that because the worker has severe degenerative disc disease and no defined work injury that his back pain in not caused by his employment.

The singularist method is another approach to causality. The singularist approach to causality is characterized by the idea that the correct definition of causal-ity must be framed in terms of one single case of causal sequence.

The American Medical Association Guides to the Evaluation of Permanent Impairment (fourth edition), defines causation as a physical, chemical or biologic factor that contributes to the occurrence of a medical condition. The fifth edition states that a factor caused or worsened a medical condition, two criteria must be verified: the factor in question could have caused on contributed to worsening of the impairment, and the factor did cause or contribute to worsening of the impairment. The fifth edition of the Guides describes causation as an identifiable factor that results in a medically identifiable condition.

Medical based causation requires a detailed analysis of whether the factor caused the condition. You need to determine if the alleged factor cause permanent impairment? Causation in civil litigation and workman's condition varies from jurisdiction to jurisdiction. You need to be aware of the definition of causation in your jurisdiction. You must be aware that multiple factors can cause an injury resulting in an impairment. You also may need to estimate the degree to which each factor contributed to a specific impairment. Some of these factors may have been present prior to a recent injury .In these cases apportionment may be used to distribute multiple factors (i.e. preexisting injury, or impairment) that caused the impairment. To determine apportionment the following must be present:

1.   A document of a prior factor.

2.   The current permanent impairment is greater as a result of the prior factor.

3.   There is reasonable probability that there is evidence that the prior factor contributed to the impairment.

Work inability or ability must also be understood. The ability for someone to work is made up of three major components: work tolerance; capacity; and risk of reinjury. The ability to tolerate discomfort or work tolerance is a dynamic blend between both physiological and non-physiological factors and cannot be scientifically measured. Work tolerance may or may not be similar to someone's current ability and is generally less than their capacity. Social and personal psychological factors can drastically influence this component thereby explaining the difference for someone to be able to work without subjective symptoms and have similar findings on examination or testing. Capacity is usually a measure of someone's current ability. Current ability can sometimes be measured scientifically, if the patient provides maximal and valid effort during a functional capacity evaluation. Many times, factors like strength, flexibility, and endurance can be increased through exercise in motivated patients. This component should be expressed according to the parameters contained in the U.S. Department of Labor's Dictionary of Occupational Titles.

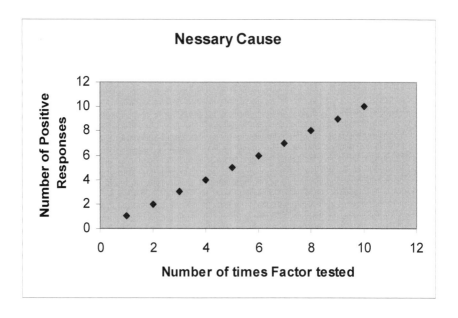

Legend for figure 2. In causation, the factor in question causes a response each time the factor occurs.

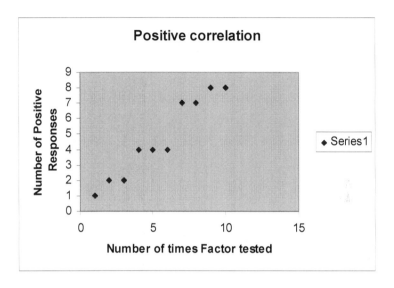

Legend for figure 3. In this example, the factor in question caused a response in a certain percentage of tests. You can not therefore state that the factor caused the event with 100% certainty.

You may want to consider the Bradford Hill model of causation to help you attempt to determine medical causation. Hills Criteria of Causation outlines the minimal conditions needed to establish a causal relationship between two items. These criteria were originally presented by Austin Bradford Hill to determine the causal link between a specific factor (e.g., cigarette smoking) and a disease (lung cancer). While it is quite easy to claim that smoking causes lung cancer, it is quite difficult when you attempt to establish a valid connection between the two events. Hill's Criteria provide an additional means to evaluate the many theories and hypotheses proposed by the claimants, adjusters, case workers, physicians etc. Professor Hill and members of the United States Public Health Department developed the following criteria which can help you to evaluate criteria to attempt to establish medical causation when two or more possible causative factors exist. Hill stated however, that cause-effect decisions cannot be based on a set of rules. Hill also stated that both the medical, scientific and legal establishments need to consider costs and benefits when making decisions about health-care interventions.

1. Temporal Relationship: Exposure always precedes the outcome. If factor "A" is believed to cause a disease, then it is clear that factor "A" must necessarily always precede the occurrence of the disease. This is the only absolutely essential criterion. If the cases presented revealed that each claimant had lumbar degenerative disc disease this makes causation determination more difficult. Degenerative disc disease may cause low back pain but not always. It is a chronic condition. This condition does not have to cause low back pain. However, lifting 40 pound boxes do not always cause low back pain either. In the RSD case, a fall preceded the disease.

2. Strength of the Association: This is defined by the size of the association as measured by appropriate statistical tests. The stronger the association, the more likely it is that the relation is causal. Some risk factors have a risk occurrence ratio defined. Cigarette smoking can cause lung cancer. An asbestos worker can develop lung cancer in some instances. However, if the worker smokes and also works with asbestos the worker has a higher incidence of developing lung cancer. Obesity, smoking and degenerative disc disease can be associated with low back pain. Which factor caused it?

3. Dose-Response Relationship: In some situations an exposure to an activity or exposure can cause significant impairment. If you attempt to lift a 500 pound weight you may suffer a disc herniation. If you keep attempting this task, your risk of injury increases. An increasing amount of exposure increases the risk. If a dose-response relationship is present, it is strong evidence for a causal relationship. However, the absence of a dose-response relationship does not rule out a causal relationship. You do not have to lift a 40 pound box to develop low back pain. A threshold may exist above which a relationship may develop.

At the same time, if a specific factor is the cause of a disease, the incidence of the disease should decline when exposure to the factor is reduced or eliminated.   In many instances, a low dose of activity can enable the body to repair simple sprains and strains and enable one's body to repair itself.

4. Consistency: The association is consistent when results are replicated in different settings using different methods. That is, if a relationship is causal, we would expect to find it consistently in different populations. Lifting a 40 pound box occasionally should occur in every group of workers to demonstrate consistency among studies.

This is why numerous experiments have to be done before meaningful statements can be made about the causal relationship between two or more events. For example, it has taken thousands of highly technical studies of the relationship between cigarette smoking and cancer before a definitive conclusion can be made that cigarette smoking increases the risk of cancer. Similarly, it would require numerous studies of the difference between ages and male and female performance of a specific task by a number of different workers under a variety of different circumstances before a conclusion could be made regarding whether an or gender difference exists in the performance of such behaviors.

If you examine the demographics of the injured workers in our case example, their data must be compared to that of the uninjured workers and to workers on other shifts, other departments etc to attempt to evaluate definite causation.

5.Plausibility: A conclusion can be assumed for which no sound evidence may exist. You may think that a certain virus causes a respiratory infection. However, there may be no conclusive evidence that any certain vector transmits the virus to your body even though a presumptive conclusion is believed to exist between a vector and a disease.

6.You may correlate that in even years that an overweight president will be elected president. The likelihood that these events are related are minimal or not plausible. On the other hand, the discovery of a correlation between population growth and the use of oil in the United States is logical and plausible.

7. Consideration of Alternate Explanations: In judging whether a factor is the cause of an event then it is necessary to determine the extent to which researchers have taken other possible causes into account and have effectively ruled out alternate explanations.

In other words, it is necessary to consider multiple hypotheses before making conclusions about relationship between any two items under investigation. This is where comparison to a placebo group is important. If factor A causes event B, then event B should not occur. If B occurs without A then other causes of B must be ruled out to state that events A and B are related.

8.Experiment: The condition can be altered by an appropriate experimental regimen. Well designed studies are discussed in the chapter that discusses evidence based medicine. You must use caution however, if you try an extrapolate animal studies with causation in humans. It would be extremely difficult to argue causation of low back pain in our case example based upon animal studies.

9.Specificity: This is established when a single cause produces a specific event. When a acidic solution contacts litmus paper, the litmus paper turns red. On the other hand, the causes attributed to lung cancer do not meet these criteria. When specificity of an association is found, it provides additional support for a causal relationship. However, absence of specificity in no way negates a causal relationship. Causality is most often multiple especially when discussing human medical conditions because multiple factors are usually involved. This is the weakest criteria when discussing injury causation or disease causation. Therefore, it is necessary to examine specific causal relationships within a larger systemic perspective to formulate a plausible conclusion.

10. Coherence: This is determined when the cause is consistent with the natural history of the effect. The association should be compatible with existing theory and current knowledge. In other words, it is necessary to evaluate claims of causality within the context of the current state of knowledge within a given field. However, as with the issue of plausibility, research that disagrees with established theory and knowledge are not automatically false. They may in fact, force a reconsideration of accepted beliefs and principles. As you can see, injury causation in general can be extremely difficult. In many instances, a court must make the decision.

One may conclude from reading this chapter that RSD/CRPS causation is difficult. One can only state that a certain event contributed to the onset of RSD/CRPS.

7.   Diagnosis of RSD/CRPS

There is minimal consensus among physicians with respect to the diagnosis of CRPS. Reflex sympathetic dystrophy (RSD) is now referred to as the Complex Regional Pain Syndrome (CRPS). Unfortunately, it is a difficult entity to diagnose and treat   CRPS was initially described by Mitchell, Morehouse, and Keen in 1864. Civil War soldiers who suffered injuries to their arms and legs developed burning pain, swelling and discoloration of their limbs following their injuries. This syndrome was called reflex sympathetic dystrophy (RSD). RSD/CRPS occurs in approximately 0.05 %-15 % of patients following extremity surgery or trauma. RSD implied a reflex mechanism associated with a hyperactive nervous system where the affected extremity swells, becomes cold and sweats profusely. The International Association changed the name for RSD for the Study of Pain (IASP) in 1994 to the Complex Regional Pain Syndrome (CRPS). If no nerve injury was identified the entity was called CRPS I. If a nerve injury was present, the term CRPS II was used.

The criteria for the diagnosis of RSD/CRPS are mainly based on the patient's history and physical examination and is determined by the patient's examining physician. There is no X ray or other tests that will diagnose RSD/CRPS. All four of the following criteria can be used for the diagnosis of RSD to be established: 1. the presence of an initiating noxious event, or a cause of immobilization; 2. continuing pain, pain with which the pain is disproportionate to the initiating event; 3. confirmation at some time of edema, changes in blood flow, or abnormal sweating activity in the area of the pain such as changes in skin temperature, skin color, or sweating; 4. and the absence of other conditions that would account for the pain and dysfunction. The International Association for the Study of Pain (IASP) criteria for RSD/CRPS suggest that for a patient to have a diagnosis of RSD/CRPS the patient should have the following: at least one patient complaint in each of the following general categories: 1.sensory: increased sensitivity to a sensory stimulation (e.g. touch), vasomotor: temperature abnormalities or skin color changes, sudomotor: sweating of the hand or foot or swelling of the hand or foot, or motor: inability to move the hand or foot, weakness or tremors of the hand or foot, and (2) at least one observable sign within two or more of the above four categories previously mentioned. One must rule out the more common conditions that could mimic RSD/CRPS such as diabetic or thyroid neuropathies, nerve entrapment syndromes such as the carpal tunnel syndrome, disc disease or the thoracic outlet syndrome. Also, one should consider in the differential diagnosis the following: deep vein thrombosis, cellulitis, vascular insufficiency, lymphedema, and erythromelalgia. The ISAP established the guidelines in order to standardize the diagnosis of RSD/CRPS.

The American Medical Association publishes the Guides to Permanent Impairment, Fifth Edition. These authors established guidelines for the diagnosis of RSD/CRPS that some clinicians feel are too stringent. These guidelines require more criteria for one to make a diagnosis of RSD. In the **AMA GUIDES TO THE EVALUATION OF PERMANENT IMPAIRMENT**, 5th Edition, on page 496, the clinical guidelines state that there "must" be at least eight (8) of 11 concurrent, objective signs for RSD in order to make the diagnosis. The AMA currently requires eight of the following criteria to diagnose RSD: the skin must be mottled, the skin temperature should be cool, there should be swelling of the foot or hand, the skin of the hand or foot should be overly moist, the skin texture should be smooth about the fingers and toes, there should be soft tissue entropy in the fingertips, stiffness of the joints of the hand or foot must be present, the length of the fingernails or toenails should be different from the hand or foot without RSD/CRPS and must be observed, the hair on the arms or legs of the affected extremity should either be longer or have fallen out, osteoporosis should be noted on x-ray, and a bone scan should be consistent with RSD. It is interesting that the **AMA GUIDES TO THE EVALUATION OF PERMANENT IMPAIRMENT**, 4th Edition, page 56 suggests the following for the diagnosis of RSD: pain, swelling, stiffness and discoloration. In the Workman's Compensation setting, some states rely on the AMA guidelines in order for one to make a diagnosis of RSD. Their insurance companies do not tell some patients that the AMA guide-lines are used to deny authorization for treatments. If you compare The ISAP Criteria for the diagnosis of RSD with the AMA guidelines, you will notice that you can have RSD by the ISAP criteria but not have RSD by the AMA criteria.

You should be aware that there is no diagnostic gold standard or an objective test for the diagnosis of RSD/CRPS. However, some diagnostic tests do add important information that may help confirm the diagnosis even though a normal result does not rule out the possibility of a RSD/CRPS diagnosis. In other words, if a doctor tells you that you do not have RSD/CRPS. based on a three-phase bone scan for example, you should realize that this individual is committing a grave error. You may indeed have this disease in spite of having a normal three-phase bone scan.

RSD is an abnormality of one's sympathetic nervous system. A test that measures blood flow in an arm or leg can help to assess your sympathetic nervous system. If the sympathetic nervous system is hyperactive, you will have a decrease in blood flow in your affected extremities. If your sympathetic nervous system is not active, you will experience an increase in blood flow in your extremities that have RSD/CRPS. RSD/CRPS is reported to be associated with a malfunction in your sympathetic nervous system (either increased activity or decreased activity). Your doctor can assess your sympathetic nervous system function using a laser Doppler or thermographic device. For example, if your sympathetic nervous system is abnormal in your right hand, you can test your hand sympathetic nervous system by putting your feet in ice water. You take a base line picture of both hands before the ice bath and immediately afterwards. Your hands should exhibit decreased blood flow. If one hand has RSD/CRPS, your blood flow will not decrease. Remember that other diseases such as a diabetic neuropathy can be associated with an abnormal sympathetic nervous system.

A three phase bone scan, MRI, skin tests, joint fluid analysis to rule our arthritis, laser Doppler fluxmetry and thermography can be used to assess sympathetic nervous system function. Remember that these tests do not diagnose RSD. Sometimes the chemical phentolamine test is used to assess sympathetic nervous system function. Reflex sympathetic dystrophy (RSD) is associated a wide range of symptoms, and except for pain, not all of the symptoms may be apparent or necessary for establishing a diagnosisaccording to the IASP criteria.

The Signs and symptoms of RSD/CRPS may be summarized as: Pain: A patient's pain is described as severe, deep, burning, and/or aching. Allodynia is pain from light touch or from a light breeze. Gently tapping the skin can cause severe pain. Motor Involvement: Decreased movement of the affected arm or leg can be detected which can be due to the tendency of the patient to guard the area of pain by restricting motion. This can lead to progressive loss or muscle mass or wasting called atrophy which can cause the limb to become fixed in one position. This is called a contracture.

Lower extremity RSD/CRPS may initially be associated with hot, swollen inflammation of the affected area characterized by increased blood flow (Phase I) and then proceed to the cold stage caused by decreased blood flow (Phase III) which is subsequently associated with muscle shrinkage of the hand or foot because the blood flow and nutritional supply are significantly reduced. Autonomic Changes: Increase or decrease of skin temperature. Cyanosis (blue skin), red, or mottled color to the patient's skin. Inflammatory/Trophic Changes: Brittle nails on the affected hand or foot which may grow faster or slower than the normal hand or foot. Hair may grow faster pr fall out on the affected extremity. Increased sweating (hyperhydrosis) is common on RSD/CRPS. Edema or swelling of the affected limb frequently occurs. A smooth, glossy appearance to skin may be seen. Patchy bone demineralization is seen on X ray in the affected extremity. If you receive denial of coverage of your RSD, ask your physician which diagnostic criteria were used to deny that you have RSD. In summary, there are no diagnostic tests to confirm the diagnosis of RSD. Be aware that the diagnosis is only be made by careful analysis of the history and clinical picture by your physician. This concept has been mentioned in this chapter multiple times and will be mentioned again and again to drive this point home.

A variety of other conditions can mimic the signs and symptoms of reflex sympathetic dystrophy and have to be ruled out before a definite diagnosis of RSD can be established. These include: Rheumatoid arthritis, gout, lumbar or cervical disk herniation, peripheral neuropathy, diabetic neuropathy, nerve entrapment syndromes, osteomyelitis, septic arthritis, thoracic outlet syndrome, cellulitis, vascular insufficiency, lymphedema, bursitis, tendonitis, patella injuries of the knee, meniscal tears of the knee, femoral/tibial injury or bone fracture. Some older physicians will tell you do not have RSD because you have a normal triple phase bone scan. Insurance companies will deny you treatment also because you have a normal scan. A normal triple phase bone scan does not rule out RSD/CRPS. Pain, tenderness, stiffness and swelling are very common after fractures and other injuries to limbs, and have a predictable time of healing. In other words, a normal injury to a bone can mimic RSD/CRPS. RSD/CRPS probably occurs in about 1 - 2% of all people who have sustained a fracture, and causalgia occurs in a slightly higher percentage of patients. In 10–20% of cases, no direct cause for RSD/CRPS is found. An injury that precedes the onset of the condition may or may not be significant with respect to RSD/CRPS causation. Other tests can be used to aid in sympathetic nervous system function. You will note that the following tests may add value to aid in the diagnosis of RSD/CRPS: Quantitative sensory testing, the quantitative sudomotor axon reflex test, and the cold presser test combined with thermographic imaging have all been used for the assessment of sympathetic nervous system function. Because these modalites are infrequently used, there will not be an in depth discussion of them. Electroneurodiagnostic sudomotor testing, the sympathetic skin response test and thermography alone have furthermore, been used to assess sympathetic nervous system activity. As stated previously, the clinical findings remain the gold standard for the diagnosis of RSD/CRPS, and the tests described above may serve as additional tools to establish the diagnosis in doubtful cases.

The degree of unilateral vascular disturbances (hot or cold skin) in RSD/CRPS depends on your sympathetic nervous system activity. Considering this, skin temperature differences in the distal arms or legs are capable of distinguishing RSD/CRPS from other extremity pain syndromes. You should be aware however, that another study demonstrated that that skin temperature and color differences between the hands, which are sometimes used to support the diagnosis of RSD/CRPS, can be produced and maintained by short-term immobility of the hand or foot. It is been postulated that there is a pathological interaction between your sympathetic nervous system and the neurons within the skin if you have RSD/CRPS. Quantitative sensory testing is used by some clinicians to aid in the diagnosis of RSD/CRPS. This includes the use of standardized psychophysical tests of the thermal, thermal pain, and vibratory thresholds to assess the function of large-fiber, myelinated small-fiber, and unmyelinated small afferent fibers. Static, dynamic allodynia, pinprick allodynia, heat and mechanical hyperalgesia, and temporal summation may be abnormal in patients with RSD/CRPS. Although no specific sensory pattern has been associated with RSD/CRPS, quantification of individual signs may provide a valuable means of documenting responses to therapy.

Autonomic nervous system function tests include infrared thermometry and thermography, the quantitative sudomotor axon reflex test (QSART), the thermoregulatory sweat test (TST), and the laser Doppler flowmetry. Infrared thermography has been used to assess skin temperature differences. A difference of more than 2.2° C between the two sides of the body suggests the diagnosis of sympathetic nervous system dysfunction. The mean temperature difference in peripheral nerve injury is 1.5°C from the uninjured nerve in the opposite extremity. Early in the RSD/CRPS disease process, the affected limb may show elevated skin temperatures while chronic stages of the disease may demonstrate lower temperatures compared to the unaffected side or normal side. These observations are a result of your blood vellel caliber. Chronic RSD/CRPS can cause a chronic decrease of the caliber of your arm or leg arteries. Vascular reflex re-sponses may be assessed using laser Doppler fluxmetry. In patients with RSD/CRPS of less than 16 weeks, the affected extremity may exhibit higher skin perfusion. In patients with a duration of the age of 15 months, the skin perfusion is either higher or lower, while in patients with a duration of RSD/CRPS of 28 months or greater, the arm or leg have lower skin temperatures. A three phase bone scan can ocasionally provide important information. Uptake in the metacarpophalangeal or metacarpal bones is thought to be suggestive for RSD/CRPS. The dark areas of the left hand below demon-strate increased isotope uptake in the left hand.

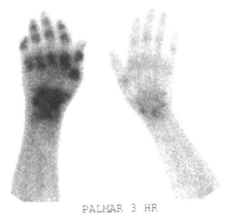

PALMAR 3 HR

Figure 1. Three phase bone scan showing uptake of the isotope into the joints and bones of the left hand.

Thermography involves the use of an infrared thermometer to measure several symmetrical points on the affected and contralateral extremity, making comparisons between the two extremities. In general, a difference of 0.5 degrees C is mildly asymmetrical, and a difference of 1.0 degrees C is considered significant. Thermographic devices portray small temperature differences between sides of the body as images. The thermographic device senses body temperature and demonstrates areas of differing heat emission by producing patterns that the physician interprets. Heat emission signals are amplified and transmitted to a monitor and/or videotape. The images may be in color or in black and white, and may be accompanied by displays of various calculations. Thermographic devices portray small temperature differences between sides of the body as images.

Another objective in doing physiologic tests is to obtain information about the involvement of the sympathetic system in RSD/CRPS. High and low whole body cooling and warming induces and reduces sympathetic vasoconstrictor activity in the hands and feet. The temperature difference between the hands in the RSD/CRPS patients increases significantly when the sympathetic system is provoked. One example of this evaluation is to place your feet in an ice bath if you have RSD/CRPS of your hand. The tem-perature of both hand should decrease if you have a normal sympathetic nervous system. If one hand has an abnormal sympathetic nervous system, your skin temperature will not decrease. Although RSD/CRPS is well documented in the extremities it has also been reported in the breast after a modified radical mastectomy. The patient had signs of RSD/CRPS and symptoms of pain, swelling, epidermal scaling, and cutaneous temperature changes lasting more than 1 year. Liquid crystal thermographic scanning revealed a significant hypothermic region in the affected breast. Intravenous phentolamine temporarily relieved the symptoms. Subsequent sympathetic blockade of the stellate ganglion alleviated chronic RSD/CRPS symptoms. Patients should be alert that RSD/CRPS needs to be considered in the differential diagnosis of chronic disproportionate pain after breast surgery.

Some researchers have advocated the use of systemic sympathetic blockade with phentolamine as a diagnostic test for RSD/CRPS. Phentolamine mesylate (Regitine) is a short-acting drug which dilates blood vessels. As a test to diagnose RSD, patients are usually given an intravenous infusion of 25 to 75 mg phentolamine for 20 minutes. Pain relief following phentolamine administration is a confirmation of sympathetic dysfunction.

There are two sub-types of RSD/CRPS. Sympathetically maintained pain is RSD/CRPS that is affected by the sympathetic nervous system. A sympathetic injection (stellate ganglion block or lumbar sympathetic block) may relieve your pain. This is called sympathetic maintained pain and your pain may be relieved by a series of sympathetic injections. RSD/CRPS pain that is not relieved by a sympathetic injection is called sympathetically independent pain. Further injections will therefore not relieve your pain.

Laser Doppler flowmetry has been used to evaluate hand and foot blood flow in patients with RSD/CRPS because it has been suggested that RSD/CRPS may be associated with blood vessel disturbances. Laser Doppler flowmetry can be used to gauge anatomical vascular mapping and capillary blood flow in the affected extremity. Investigators assessed the role of the sympathetic nervous system in patients with RSD of the hand using laser Doppler flowmetry. Cutaneous blood flow, skin resistance and skin temperature were measured at the RSD/CRPS affected and normal hands. These investigators found that differences in skin temperature and blood flow are dynamic values depending critically on environmental temperature. Sympathetic dysfunction is regularly seen at the onset of RSD/CRPS and normalizes during the course of the disease. This temporary phenomenon suggests that a posttraumatic sympathetic deficit plays a decisive role in the genesis of RSD/CRPS. Complex regional pain syndrome type I (CRPS I) is a frequent complication after injuries of the upper limbs. The pathophysiology of this disease remains unclear, although disturbances of the sympathetic nervous system have been detected in several clinical studies, and sympathetic blocks resolve the symptoms in many of the cases.

RSD/CRPS research continues. To investigate the meaning of sympathetic dysfunction at the beginning of RSD/CRPS, patients with distal radial fracture were examined prospectively during the course of the disease with regard to their clinical symptoms and their peripheral sympathetic nervous function. Sympathetic nervous function was examined by testing the vasoconstrictor response to sympathetic stimuli recorded with laser Doppler fluxmetry of the fingertips of both hands. Fracture patients revealed slightly impaired sympathetic nervous function on the first posttraumatic day and normal results during the rest of the observation time. RSD/CRPS patients had abnormal sympathetic function for the duration of the study. With regard to the unaffected opposite hand, RSD/CRPS patients showed impaired sympathetic nervous system function. The results of this study suggest that the disturbances in the sympathetic nervous system in RSD/CRPS patients are systemic and not limited to the affected limb. Their occurrence before the clinical breakout of the disease may serve as a marker that might be useful for early therapy and lead to further understanding of the pathophysiology of RSD/CRPS.

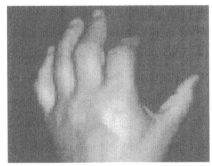 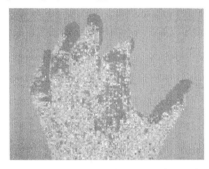

Legend for figure 2. Laser Doppler study. The swollen hand on the left picture is early RSD/CRPS. The right sided picture is a laser Doppler imagethat shows increased blood flow in the fingers of the hand.

Vascular disturbances in RSD/CRPS are not due to constant overactivity of sympathetic neurons according to some researchers. Changes in vascular sensitivity to cold temperature and circulating catecholamines (chemicals that can increase your heart rate and constrict your blood vessels) may be responsible for blood vessel abnormalities and not to an overactive nervous system. On the other hand, RSD/CRPS may be associated with an abnormal reflex pattern of sympathetic vasoconstrictor neurons due to thermoregulatory and emotional stimuli generated in the central nervous system (brain and spinal cord). Other investigators compared several types of imaging studies for the purpose of diagnosing post traumatic RSD/CRPS. In one study, 158 patients with distal forearm fractures were followed for 16 weeks after sustaining fractures. A detailed clinical examination was carried out 2, 8, and 16 weeks after trauma by a physician in conjunction with bilateral thermography, plain radiographs of the hand, 3-phase bone scan, and magnetic resonance imaging (MRI). These results suggested that those diagnostic modalities can not be used as screening tests. Imaging methods are not able to reliably differentiate between normal post-traumatic changes and changes due to RSD/CRPS. Clinical findings as previously stated remain the gold standard for the diagnosis of RSD/CRPS and the procedures described above may serve as only additional tools to establish the diagnosis in doubtful cases.

Patients with RSD/CRPS may have temperature differences between the extremity with RSD/CRPS and the extremity that does not have RSD/CRPS. If you have RSD/CRPS your normal hand or foot be warmer or cooler than the RSD/CRPS hand or foot. You can measure the temperature of your skin with an infrared skin surface monitor. Thermographic recordings of the palmar/plantar side and dorsal side of both hands or feet were made on RSD /CRPS patients and in control fracture patients with and without and without patient complaints similar to RSD/CRPS in one study. The RSD/CRPS involved side in RSD/CRPS patients was warmer compared with the non-involved extremity. The difference in temperature between the involved site and the non-involved extremity in RSD/CRPS patients significantly differed from the difference in temperature between the opposite extremities of the 2 control groups. The largest temperature difference between extremities was found in RSD/CRPS patients. These investigators concluded that the validity of skin surface temperature recordings under resting conditions to discriminate between acute RSD/CRPS1 fracture patients and control fracture patients with/without complaints is limited.

It can be concluded from reading this chapter that no specific diagnostic test is available for the diagnosis of RSD/CRPS. As a result, the diagnosis of RSD/CRPS is based primarily on a patient's history, the clinical examination, and any supportive laboratory findings only.

8. Epidemiology of RSD/CRPS

You should know the epidemiology of RSD/CRPS in order to better understand this disease. Epidemiology is the study of diseases in a certain population. To be more specific, epidemiology is the study of factors affecting the health of specific populations, and serves as the foundation for interventions made in the interest of public health. Prevalence is defined as the total number of cases of the disease in the population at a given time. Incidence is a measure of the risk of developing some new condition within a specified period of time. Before giving the epidemiology of RSD/CRPS, epidemiologists must rule out other diseases that can mimic RSD. This process is called making a differential diagnosis. The differential diagnosis of RSD/CRPS includes infection, neuropathies, factitious disorder, a conversion reaction, rheumatologic disorders, vascular disorders and a blood vessel infection. RSD/CRPS should be distinguished from neuralgia. Neuralgia causes paroxysmal pain usually confined to one nerve distribution as opposed to the constant burning pain that does not follow the distribution of a nerve. Blood vessel, muscle and sweat changes are usually not seen with neuralgia.

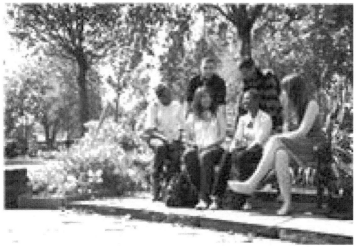

Figure 1. Epidemiology is the study of diseases in a certain population. To be more specific, epidemiology is the study of factors affecting the

health of specific populations, and serves as the foundation for interventions made in the interest of public health.

RSD/CRPS Epidemiology

Average Age (years) 41.8

GenderFemale to Male 3:1

Location of RSD/CRPS 44 % upper extremity

48 % lower extremity

Injury type 29 % sprain/strain of arm or leg

24 % post surgical

11 % contusion or crush injury

RSD/CRPS: Prevalence and Occupation

14 %   Service occupations (restaurant workers, bakers, police etc.)

8 %   Clerical/sales

7.4 % Manual labor

5.2 % Professional, technical, managerial

5.2 % Agricultural, fishing, forestry

4.4 % Bench work

2.2 % Machine trades

4.4 % Bus drivers/truck drivers

5 %   Occupation not determined

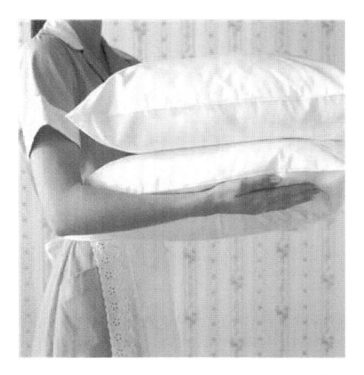

Figure 2. Individuals in a service occupation are more prone to develop RSD/CRPS.

The upper limb is affected by RSD/CRPS more commonly than the lower limb. Approximately 10.7% of RSD/CRPS cases noted in a previous epidemiologic study were noted to be non-traumatic. In 89.3% of the patients, RSD/CRPS developed after a traumatic inciting event with a predominance of fractures. In 75.6% of patients, RSD/CRPS developed due to occupational injuries. The percentage of successful clinical outcome was 72%. The percentage of the patients that did not respond to therapy was 28%. The management period is long and this causes higher therapeutic costs in addition to loss of job productivity. However, overall, the response to therapy is good. On the other hand, in approximately one third of the patients, RSD/CRPS does not improve despite all therapeutic interventions.

Many patients suffering from RSD/CRPS are not seen by a RSD/CRPS specialist in a timely fashion. It has been reported that with respect to RSD/CRPS in general, patients had seen on average 4.8 different physicians before referral to a pain center and had received an average of five different kinds of treatments both prior to and during pain clinic treatment. The mean duration of RSD/CRPS symptoms prior to a pain center evaluation was 30 months. Seventeen percent had a lawsuit and 54% had a workman's compensation claim related to the RSD/CRPS.

Fifty-one of the patients in this study received a bone scan, but only 53% of the bone scans were interpreted as consistent with the diagnosis of RSD/CRPS. Forty-seven percent had a history of physician-imposed immobilization, and 56% had a myofascial component present at evaluation. The duration of RSD/CRPS symptoms and the involvement of the upper extremity were significantly associated with the presence of myofascial dysfunction. Unfortunately, most CRPS/RSD patients are referred to a pain specialty clinic after several years of symptoms and many failed therapies. The data also suggest the lack of utility of a diagnostic bone scan and highlight the prominence of myofascial dysfunction in a majority of RSD/CRPS patients. The incidence of RSD/CRPS type I is higher than RSD/CRPS type II. The reported incidence of RSD/CRPS type II is 1-2% after various fractures , while the incidence of RSD/CRPS type I approximates 1-5% after peripheral nerve injury. The incidence of RSD/CRPS is 12% after brain trauma and 5% after a heart attack.

The incidence of RSD/CRPS both type 1 & 2 are about 1% to 15% overall. There appears to be higher occurrence of RSD/CRPS in females. The ratio of female: male is 3:1. (3) The affected age group is between 18 and 71 years with a mean age of 41.8 years. RSD/CRPS can also occur in children. Children with diabetes have highest incidence of RSD/CRPS as compared to non-diabetic children. Past research indicates several causes linking to the disease. The most common is being trauma. The severity of trauma may range from sprain to gunshot wound. There is no correlation between the severities of insult to the severity of the RSD/CRPS. Other causes are venipuncture, infection; surgery, arthritis, coronary artery disease, Parkinson's disease, head injury, burns, dental extractions and stroke. However, in a large number of cases it is hard to find any cause.

There are several risks factors that have been identified for RSD/CRPS; among them are immobilization of an arm or leg following injury, smoking, substance abuse, genetic, and psychological factors. Immobilization for prolonged periods of time of an injured limb could cause development of RSD/CRPS. Smoking is also considered as a potential risk factor. There is a higher percentage (30%) of substance abuse among patients with RSD/CRPS.

One retrospective study reveals a higher incidence of premorbid history of depression and anxiety disorder in RSD/CRPS patients. Although many studies fail to provide any specific personality factors for the development of RSD/CRPS it has been suggested that patients with dependent personalities and those who have problems with authority and slow promotion rates have higher incidences of RSD/CRPS. With respect to litigation, 95 patients have been previously studied. Twenty-three (17%) of these patients' medical records reflected either current or a previous involvement in a lawsuit in relationship to their RSD/CRPS. Seventy-two (54%) of the patients had a workerman's compensation claim related to their RSD/CRPS. Twenty-three percent of the patients reported having undergone an independent medical examination at some point at the request of legal or worker's compensation authorities.

The season of the year may be associated with the onset of RSD/CRPS. The season of the year in which the injury occurred leading to the development of RSD/CRPS occurred can be taken into consideration in the etiology of RSD. Injuries appeared to be slightly more common during the summer months (27%) as compared with injuries occurring in winter (21%), spring (24%) and fall (19%). Thirty-eight percent of patients reportedly had a report of receiving a bone scan prior to or following their evaluation at a pain clinic. Of these patients with a clinical diagnosis of RSD, 53% were officially interpreted by the performing radiologist as having findings consistent with RSD while 47% had a negative bone scan interpreted as not consistent with the diagnosis of RSD.

Patients prior admission to a pain clinic had been prescribed 5.2 (range, 2 to 8) different kinds of treatments, ranging from various medications to more aggressive treatment such as spinal cord stimulators. The majority of patients had received antidepressant medications. Specifically 78% of patients had received tricyclic antidepressants (amitriptyline) and 38% had received selective serotonin reuptake inhibitors (Zoloft). It would be important if these antidepressants were prescribed for pain, sleep, or psychiatric disorders. Other pharmacologic agents patients received included anticonvulsant drugs (60%) and opiate (70%) drugs. Non-pharmacologic therapies included physical therapy (88%), occupational therapy (45%) and psychotherapy (50%). Nerve blocks had been given to 82% of patients with the mean number of nerve blocks being six. The vast majority of nerve blocks were performed prior to pain center treatment. Eight patients (6%) had a spinal cord stimulator implanted to relieve their symptoms of RSD/CRPS.

Immobilization of an arm or leg can be associated with the development of RSD. Immobilization is frequently done following the extremity injury with a cast or splint. Another form of immobilization is patient imposed restricted movement due to pain and guarding. In other words if your arm or leg hurts with movement, you may resist any movement. Fifty-six percent of the patients had a documented muscle pain component associated with RSD/CRPS, based on the physician's examination for trigger points. Trigger points are areas of muscle tenderness that cause a wide spread pattern of pain when pressed on by the examining physician or therapist. The presence or absence of a muscle component was determined by palpating for muscle trigger points in the patient's musculature. When trigger points were present they reproduced some or all of the patient's RSD/CRPS symptoms.

Muscle pain (called myofascial pain) is frequently seen in patients with RSD as was mentioned above. The incidence of myofascial pain is greater in upper extremity RSD/CRPS as opposed to lower extremity RSD. In addition, the longer the duration of RSD/CRPS symptoms the more likely a patient was to exhibit a myofascial component. The mean duration of symptoms in patients with the presence of myofascial trigger points was 35 months and those without myofascial trigger points were 23 months.

You should now be aware that only minimal information has been published regarding the epidemiology of RSD/CRPS. Besides having an unknown pathophysiology, scant information is available describing the types of patients that develop RSD/CRPS and the types of health care services rendered to treat this disorder. Most patients with RSD/CRPS are Caucasian. It has been hypothesized that there may be a genetic predisposition to the development of RSD following bodily injury. Aggressive early treatment improves outcome. Most RSD pain clinic referrals come from surgeons. Only few patients are referred by primary care physicians. Remember that a delay in the proper diagnosis and treatment of RSD/CRPS may have a negative effect on patient outcome. In other words, a timely diagnosis and the prompt initiation of treatment will improve patient outcome. The use of nerve blocks reflects a physicians' outdated training. For example, the classical teaching is that RSD/CRPS was treated with sympathetic nerve blockade. Now it is known that the proper treatment is a multidisciplinary approach which minimizes the role of sympathetic blocks.

The presence of worker compensation and litigation issues is felt to be common in many chronic pain conditions that frequently are associated with job related injuries. The relatively high frequency of work related accidents that are associated with the development of RSD/CRPS is not unexpected because the most frequent cause of this condition is a traumatic injury. It is interesting to attempt to identify the types of jobs RSD/CRPS patients had when injured. Service occupations, such as restaurant workers and police officers, suffered almost twice as often from RSD/CRPS as other occupations. Manual laborers were the next highest group. The increased incidence of RSD/CRPS in these groups is likely due to the physical demands related to these jobs.

It is furthermore, interesting to note that RSD/CRPS patients who had received a three phase bone scan only 53% had a positive test. This finding should seriously question the clinical utility of the three phase bone scan in the diagnosis of RSD/CRPS. The three phase bone scan's role in clinical practice needs to be justified because of the expense involved. Immobilization may suggest that immobilization of a limb may play a role in the origin of RSD/CRPS. Animal studies have demonstrated that immobilizing a rodent limb results in the development of RSD/CRPS signs and symptoms. Additionally, changes in the rat spinal cord are similar to that seen in experimental rat peripheral nerve injuries. Furthermore, a clinical study found that signs and symptoms of RSD/CRPS develop in casted orthopedic patients following uncomplicated surgery. Physicians and patients therefore, need to be educated on the importance of early and gradual mobilization following soft-tissue injury, especially following surgery or trauma.

Based on the finding that the duration of RSD/CRPS is associated with the presence of clinically relevant trigger points, it may be assumed that muscle dysfunction develops secondarily over time due to pain and disuse of the involved limb. Physicians should evaluate RSD/CRPS patients for the presence of muscle trigger points and treat appropriately when present with physical therapy and other modalities such as trigger points.

In conclusion, this chapter has described the epidemiology and health care utilization of RSD/CRPS patients. Multiple consultations and therapies are obtained by these patients. In addition, a substantial percentage of these patients have a history of limb immobilization and a significant muscle pain component identified on initial evaluation.

9. Psychological Effects and Pain

Patients with RSD/CRPS can develop psychological pathology following the onset of their disease because of his/her disability and severe pain. Their severe pain can cause anxiety and patients may develop pain-induced depression. Psychological illness prior to the onset of RSD/CRPS can be associated with pain manifestations as well. The following findings relate to how an individual's psychological state influences his or her perception of and response to pain: Patients who have strongly negative emotions about a situation experience more pain. Women have more negative emotions about situations in general than men and, therefore, have a higher incidence of pain. However, women cope better with pain than men. Family members' and friends' pain may influence an individual's own pain. For example, women whose immediate family members were experiencing significant pain experienced more clinical pain and complained of more severe pain themselves. In general, men do not demonstrate this effect.

The most common personality disorders are the somatoform disorders. The somatoform disorders are a group of mental disturbances that are diagnosed on the basis of their symptoms. These disorders are characterized by physical complaints that appear to be medical in origin but that cannot be explained in terms of a physical disease. Pseudodysyrophy can occur in patients which is not RSD/CRPS. Pseudodystrophy and reflex sympathetic dystrophy, although sharing some similar clinical features, can be distinguished as two different conditions, each requiring its own approach and management. The most important distinction is found on bone scintigraphy. In reflex sympathetic dystrophy the bone scan shows a typical increased tracer uptake (at least during stages I and II); in pseudodystrophy there is a normal or decreased tracer uptake in the affected region. Moreover the vascularization is increased in reflex sympathetic dystrophy stage I, whereas in pseudodystrophy hypovascularization is found from the beginning. The physical symptoms must be serious enough to interfere with a patient's employment or relationships, and must not be under the patient's voluntary control in order to qualify as a somatoform disorder. In general, the somatoform disorders are characterized by disturbances in the patient's physical sensations or ability to move the limbs or walk, while the dissociative disorders are marked by disturbances in the patient's sense of identity or memory.

The somatoform disorders are difficult to recognize and treat because patients often have long histories of medical or surgical treatment with several different doctors. In addition, the physical symptoms are not under the patient's conscious control, so that he or she is not intentionally trying to confuse the doctor or complicate the process of diagnosis. Somatoform disorders are a significant problem for the health care system because these patients overuse medical services and resources. A somatoform disorder that can be difficult to treat is the somatization disorder. The somatization disorder was formerly called Briquet's syndrome, after the French physician who first recognized it. The distinguishing characteristic of this disorder is a group or pattern of symptoms in several different organ systems of the patient's body that cannot be ascertained by a medical illness.

The diagnosis of the somatization disorder requires four symptoms of pain, two symptoms in the digestive tract, one symptom involving the sexual organs, and one symptom related to the nervous system. The somatization disorder usually begins before the age of 30. It is estimated that 0.2% of the United States population will develop this disorder in the course of their lives. The female-to-male ratio is estimated to range between 5:1 and 20:1. The somatization disorder is considered a chronic disturbance that tends to persist throughout the patient's life. It usually begins in the teenage years. It is also likely to run in families. A conversion disorder may be suspected in individuals who experience a loss of sensation without a medical cause.

A conversion disorder is a condition in which the patient's senses or ability to walk or move are impaired without a recognized medical or neurological disease or cause and in which psychological factors such as stress or trauma are the causes of this disorder. In this disorder, the patient is converting a psychological conflict or problem into an inability to move specific parts of the body or to use the senses normally. A conversion reaction contains the anxiety and serves to get the patient out of the threatening situation. The resolution of the emotion that underlies the physical symptom is called the patient's primary gain, and the change in the patient's social, occupational, or family situation that results from the symptom is called a secondary gain. Some physical symptoms of a conversion disorder include a loss of balance, paralysis of an arm or leg, the inability to swallow or speak; the loss of touch or pain sensation; loss of sight or hearing, double vision or having seizures. Unlike the somatization disorder, a conversion disorder may begin at any age, and it does not appear to run in families. A conversion disorder usually occurs among less educated or sophisticated people. A conversion disorder is not usually a chronic disturbance. The female-to-male ratio is 2:1. Male patients are likely to develop conversion disorders in occupational settings or military service.

Another personality disorder is the pain disorder. The pain disorder is noted by the presence of severe pain as the patient's focus. This category of somatoform disorder covers a range of patients with a variety of ailments, including chronic headaches, back problems, arthritis, muscle aches and cramps, or pelvic pain. In some cases the patient's pain appears to be largely due to psychological factors, but in other cases the pain is derived from a medical condition as well as the patient's psychology. This disorder is seen in older patients.

Hypochondrias is a somatoform disorder marked by excessive fear of or preoccupation with having a serious illness that persists in spite of negative medical testing. Hypochondriasis is usually seen in young adults. Flare-ups of this disorder are often correlated with stressful events in the patient's life. Both the somatization disorder and hypochondriasis may result from the patient's unconscious reflection or imitation of parental behaviors. This behavior is particularly likely if the patient's parent derived considerable secondary gain from his or her symptoms. An accurate diagnosis of somatoform disorders is important to prevent unnecessary pain procedures, surgery, laboratory tests, or other treatments and procedures. The diagnosis of somatoform disorders requires a thorough physical workup to exclude medical and neurological conditions as a cause of a pain disorder. A detailed examination is necessary when conversion disorder is a possible diagnosis.

In addition to anxiety or personality disorders, the doctor must consider major depression as a possible additional diagnosis when evaluating a patient with symptoms of a somatoform disorder. Because patients with somatoform disorders often have lengthy medical histories, a long-term relationship with a primary care practitioner can prevent unnecessary treatments. to specialists to a minimum. Patients with somatoform disorders may be treated with antianxiety drugs or antidepressant drugs. The treatment should be directed to symptom reduction and stabilization of the patient's personality.

Another psychological disorder seen in the pain patient population is the factitious disorder. Factitious disorders are a group of mental disturbances in which patients intentionally act physically or mentally ill without obvious benefits. The name factitious comes from a Latin word that means artificial. These disorders are not malingering. Patients with factitious disorders exaggerate the symptoms of a physical or mental illness by a variety of methods, including contaminating urine samples with blood, taking hallucinogens or injecting themselves with bacteria. These disorders are more common in men than in women. The Munchausen syndrome refers to patients whose factitious symptoms are dramatized and exaggerated. Many persons with Munchausen undergo major surgery repeatedly. These patients have a pathological desire to be sick. Patients with somatoform disorders believe that they have a physical disease. These individuals are not malingers. Malingering is a deliberate behavior for a known external purpose. It is not considered a form of mental illness or psychopathology. A malinger may have valid symptoms but is dishonest as to the source of the problems. For example, an individual may have sustained a disc herniation from a fall at home but claimed that it happened at work to be able to get compensation. An injury that resulted from an automobile accident may be exaggerated for financial gain. Examples include months of chiropractic treatment for low back pain, or physical therapy without improvement. This is not to be confused with those patients who have legitimate serious injuries that fail to respond to conservative treatment. There is usually a marked discrepancy between the person's claimed symptoms and the medical findings in a malingerer. Psychological disturbances ranging from anxiety to mood swings to sadness and depression are an all too familiar byproduct of the Complex Regional Pain Syndrome (RSD/CRPS). This is due in part to the disorder's mysterious and difficult-to-treat nature. Often, RSD/CRPS patients feel a loss of control from both physical and psychological perspectives. Compounding the problem, RSD/CRPS frequently is misunderstood by medical providers, friends and family members. This lack of understanding and support from others can contribute to feelings of isolation, loneliness and general distress. This is why it's important to find a health care provider who understands RSD/CRPS and who works with a team that includes a psychologist or counselor.

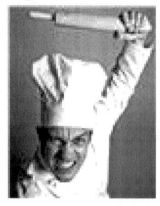

Figure 1. Psychological disturbances ranging from anxiety to mood swings to sadness and depression are an all too familiar byproduct of a Complex Regional Pain Syndrome (RSD/CRPS).

Psychological and behavioral factors can exacerbate the pain and dysfunction associated with complex regional pain syndrome (RSD/CRPS) and could help maintain the condition in some patients. Effective management of RSD/CRPS requires that these psychosocial and behavioral aspects be addressed as part of an integrated multidisciplinary treatment approach. Because emotional factors can affect pain perception and intensity, a pain specialist's complete assessment of pain should include not only a physical examination but also analysis of the psychological, emotional, and behavioral aspects of pain. Such analysis may prove challenging because many patients are reluctant to discuss painful psychological issues with their pain-management doctor (and it is more socially acceptable to seek medical rather than psychiatric care).

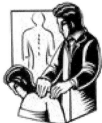

Figure 2. Sometimes consultation with a psychologist can help decrease the pain associated with RSD/CRPS by learning coping skills.

The purpose of "behavioral medicine" is to relieve anxiety and depression and to decrease pain intensity. Techniques used include biofeedback, relaxation training, and hypnosis. Because anxiety and depression can make people less able to cope with persistent pain, consultation with a behavioral medicine specialist can prove extremely beneficial. Sadness, hopelessness, insomnia, and feelings of worthlessness are all associated with depression. Anxiety is characterized by apprehension and fear or a sense of doom. Doctors need to recognize the stressors that are causing anxiety and address them with their patients. Signs and symptoms of anxiety include loss of appetite, diarrhea, fainting, increased heart rate, and sexual dysfunction.

Personality greatly influences an individual's response to pain and his or her chosen coping strategies. In general, people who have underlying anxiety are more likely to seek higher doses of pain medications. Understanding how people cope with stress is helpful; this is a task aided by discussion with the patient's family. A psychological history should include questions about depression, sleep disruption, preoccupation with body pain, reduced "everyday activities," fatigue, and loss of sexual interest. People with "psychogenic" pain make illness and hospitalization a primary goal. Psychological stresses such as anxiety and depression make pain more intense and less tolerable.

Psychologists have analyzed pre-injury personalities to identify types of people who may be more likely to develop pain syndromes. These studies conclude that there does not appear to be an unstable personality that predisposes to reflex sympathetic dystrophy or other chronic pain syndromes. Reflex sympathetic dystrophy, an extremely painful nervous system condition, was once thought to be caused by psychological disorders. According to psychological studies made after reflex sympathetic dystrophy and similar types of neuropathic (nerve injury) pain syndromes have resolved, a predisposing psychological factor is rarely associated with the pain syndrome. In some instances, however, a person's psychological makeup may control his or her sympathetic nervous system. In 1964, the behavioral aspects of seven patients' chronic reflex sympathetic dystrophy involving an extremity were reported. In each of these seven cases, financial compensation was the main motivating factor, for which these seven individuals maintained signs and symptoms of reflex sympathetic dystrophy, including each individual's chronic disability. Anxiety over potential long-term disability can actually lead to a disability in some patients. As you can see, psychological factors can affect the length of time one experiences a painful syndrome.

All patients with chronic RSD/CRPS should receive a thorough psychological evaluation, followed by cognitive-behavioral pain management treatment, including relaxation training with biofeedback. Patients making insufficient overall treatment progress or in whom co morbid psychiatric disorders/major ongoing life stressors are identified should additionally receive general cognitive-behavioral therapy to address these issues. The psychological component of treatment can work synergistically with medical and physical/occupational therapies to improve function and increase patients' ability to manage the condition successfully. Stressful life events are more common in RSD/CRPS patients. This observation indicates that there may be a multiconditional model of RSD/CRPS. The experience of stressful life events besides trauma or surgery are risk factors, not causes, in such a model.

As is the case with any chronic neuropathic pain, and particularly with RSD/CRPS, negative emotions often worsen and heighten the sensation of pain. The RSD/CRPS patient's emotions may directly activate the damaged or diseased nerves causing increases in pain perception. Therefore, it is very important for you to learn to control your emotions in response to the pain itself and to the difficulties that your chronic pain condition creates for you. There are several good techniques that will help you keep your emotions in check from further aggravating your chronic pain condition..

Many psychological pain treatments are psychological in nature. Most are fairly simple and do not require in-depth or long-term counseling. Examples include biofeedback, relaxation training, yoga and clinical hypnosis. The precise ways in which these techniques work for pain management are unknown, but patients frequently report less suffering and an improved ability to cope with chronic pain conditions such as RSD/CRPS. These modalities may be effective by lessening the number of pain signals that enter the pain center in your cortex of your brain. These simple techniques can be used in individual, group or even educational sessions. More intensive individual counseling and/or the use of prescription drugs may be required for more severe and troubling emotional problems. For example, crisis intervention for catastrophic events such as an impending divorce, loss of a job or loss of health insurance coverage can be a critical part of RSD/CRPS management. Prescription drugs may be indicated for clinical problems such as severe and persistent sleep disturbances, panic attacks, anxiety or severe depression.

Both the patient and the doctor need to identify situations that reinforce pain behavior. Patients can use a pain diary to help identify what behavior signals pain, and a family conference may help to identify the positive reinforcements (rewards) of pain, such as a doting spouse, being excused from household chores, and so on. Some people appreciate extra attention given them by family members, attention that perhaps was not available before the painful condition. Others use pain to avoid psychologically painful situations, such as workplace problems with co-workers or a supervisor, and use it to avoid going to work and dealing with colleagues. People may also use pain to avoid social or family gatherings.

Mental health specialists vary considerably in their level of training and their experience in helping patients with chronic pain. Here are some questions you can ask to find out a professional's qualifications in helping you with emotional problems that frequently accompany pain: Does your doctor belong to a recognized professional pain society, such as the American Pain Society or the American Academy of Pain Medicine? This indicates a commitment to learning about pain. If the mental health specialist is a psychiatrist (a medical doctor with special training in evaluating and treating emotional disorders) he/she can prescribe medications that can alleviate depression and anxiety.

Pain patient behaviors that should be closely watched include frequently talking about pain, moaning, and frequently going to doctors and refusing to work. Doctors should observe and note blatant pain manifestations. Pain behavior is influenced by environmental consequences. Suffering is the conceptual component of pain that denotes a persistent negative affect. Suffering is composed of depression, fear, and isolation. RSD/CRPS patients often become depressed and anxious because of chronic pain and reduced physical ability. Counseling, support groups, and chronic pain center programs can help patients learn coping strategies and can provide emotional and psychological support.

Biofeedback is often used by psychologists to treat RSD/CRPS. This intervention is effective for the reduction of pain in RSD/CRPS patients even in patients who had failed prior treatments. Changes in blood flow often accompany RSD/CRPS. Learning deep relaxation techniques can be paired with a biofeedback device which measures skin temperature in order to help a RSD/CRPS sufferer learn to relax deeply, increase blood flow to a part of the body with a restriction in blood flow, increase the temperature of that part of the body, and decrease the pain.

It is your choice as to which of these psychological methods could work best for you with respect to your pain management. Years ago, Voltaire summarized our current situation with respect to RSD/CRPS. "Doctors pour drugs, of which they know little, for disease, of which they know less, into patients, of which they know nothing." Remember that you need to receive treatment (drug or non drug) as an individual as opposed to only a pain symptom. In other words treatment must be tailored to your pathological state. The "one size fits all" philosophy must not be used in pain management. It may be concluded therefore, that behavioral medicine in many patients is an important modality for the treatment of RSD/CRPS.

10. Fibromyalgia and RSD/CRPS

Fibromyalgia is a chronic pain syndrome that affects muscles, tendons, and fascia (a tissue area over your muscle) throughout your body. This disease is also referred to as fibromyositis. It affects about 5 percent of the population, 90 percent of which are women of childbearing age. You and your physician must function together as a team to properly treat this entity. Fibromyalgia causes you to have muscle pain throughout your body, and is associated with joint stiffness and fatigue. RSD/CRPS is a disease that affects nerves, muscles and tendons.

You also may experience sleep disturbances and depression if you have fibromyalgia. It can cause many places on your body to become extremely tender. You are only diagnosed with fibromyalgia after other pain-causing conditions have been eliminated as the reason for your pain. Fibromyalgia is a condition that can be painful, but it is benign and will rarely cause you to be totally disabled. Only you can let it become disabling.

The diagnosis of fibromyalgia includes a history of aches, pains, stiffness in 11 or more tender areas above and below your navel and to the right and left of your navel (figure 1). You may have a history of irritable bowel syndrome and depression as well. You may be depressed and suffer from sleep deprivation in addition to muscle pain. The following diagram shows common body sites where you might experience tender areas associated with fibromyalgia. You muscle will not feel contracted but will feel soft and tender to light touch. Tender areas can also occur in your arms and legs. You should note from the diagram below that these tender points occur above and below your navel and occur in a plane to the right and left of your navel.

You may also suffer from myofascial pain along with your RSD/CRPS which will discussed in the next chapter. With fibromyalgia, your pain will be on both sides of your body. On the other hand, myofascial pain is frequently on one side of your body. Furthermore, RSD/CRPS begins on one side of your body, but unfortunately, this dread disease may spread to all od your extremities.

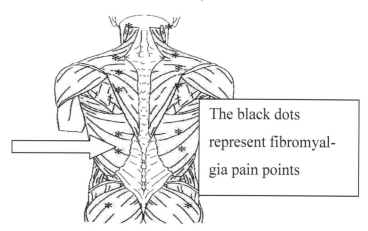

The black dots represent fibromyalgia pain points

Figure 1. There are common areas of tender points that can be associated with fibromyalgia. Note that the black dots are symmetric and represent fibromyalgia pain points.

If you are like other patients with fibromyalgia, the muscle pain that you experience is probably more common in your neck and lower back. However, it can affect any muscle throughout your body. Your pain can range from sharp or cramping to a burning sensation. Your pain may be worse in one specific area, even though the pain can be felt all over your body. You also will notice that fibromyalgia pain affects tender areas on your body that are symmetrical, or located in the same places on the opposite side of your body. Tenderness and swelling of your hands or feet are also common. Other common areas where you may notice tenderness include the areas under the base of your skull; above the shoulder blade, elbows, the buttocks (gluteal muscle); the front of the neck midway from the chin to the collar bone; the chest; the sides of the body over the hip regions; and the inner aspects of the knees.

It is more common for women to have fibromyalgia than men. Because of this, researchers are trying to find gender-specific causes of fibromyalgia. In general the amount of pain that women can withstand is lower than the amount of pain that men can withstand. Fibromyalgia is seen mostly in women between 20 and 50 years of age. However, it can affect children and elderly people as well. Fibromyalgia may develop after an injury, a motor vehicle accident, infection (viral or bacterial), or after an onset of rheumatoid arthritis. Stressful situations, cold weather and over exertion can worsen your fibromyalgia. As a fibromyalgia sufferer, you may not be getting enough deep sleep. Even in normal people, not getting enough sleep can produce symptoms of fibromyalgia. It is not currently known if a lack of deep sleep is a cause of fibromyalgia. Some doctors think the loss of deep sleep can hasten the onset of fibromyalgia.

Serotonin and norepinepherine are two chemicals in your central nervous system (brain and spinal cord) that decrease pain signals that travel to your brain. Not having enough serotonin in your brain and spinal cord can cause you lose sleep, which can cause symptoms of depression as well as fibromyalgia like pain. Fibromyalgia also affects your levels of norepinepherine, which is another chemical in your central nervous that also modulates the number of pain signals that go to your brain. Another chemical in your body that causes pain is substance P. Substance P is found in all of the neurons of your central nervous system as well as nerves that go to your muscles and joints.

When your muscle tissues have been injured, substance P is released. This event can trigger burning pain sensations throughout your body. High substance P levels have been noted in the spinal fluid of patients with fibromyalgia. Endorphins, substances produced by your body and deposited in the spinal cord to decrease pain transmission to your brain, are known to slow down the pain-causing effects of substance P. The low levels of endorphins in your brain and spinal cord when you have fibromyalgia may be another cause of pain associated with this condition.

It is well known that vigorous exercise can produce endorphins that are then released in your body. Along with decreasing the pain signals that are sent to your brain, endorphins can affect your mood. It is thought that a lower than normal blood level of endorphins may be another cause of fibromyalgia. People with and without fibromyalgia who do physical exercise have noted a decrease in their pain following aerobic exercise. Normal people usually have an increase in endorphins in their bloodstream following exercise. However, you may show no increase in endorphin levels after you exercise. There is increased evidence that fibromyalgia can be genetically inherited. You may even know of a relative who has symptoms similar to yours. The exact gene that causes fibromyalgia has not been isolated, but several genes have been proposed as a possible explanation for the genetic inheritance of fibromyalgia and they are being studied. Research into the causes of fibromyalgia must continue.

It is a good idea for you to keep a daily diary of your activities and pain levels. When you visit your doctor, be sure to take your diary with you so your doctor can see your daily activities such as exercise, sleep, and eating habits. Also be sure to write down any medications you have taken and what their effects were. This will help your doctor determine what areas you need help in the most, and can help the doctor prescribe an effective treatment to relieve your pain symptoms. Let your pain-management doctor know if your primary care doctor diagnosed any new disorder or prescribed any new drug since your last visit with your pain doctor.

It is important that you do exercise or some type of low-impact aerobic activity. Aerobic exercise is extremely helpful in decreasing your pain and improving your sleep pattern. Swimming and water aerobics are excellent ways for you to accomplish this goal. They are some of the best exercise activities for patients with fibromyalgia. These types of nonimpact activities will help strengthen and condition your muscles, unlike high-impact exercise that can actually do more damage to your muscles. A study published in 1996 said that following physical exercise, almost 50 percent of people had a significant decrease in their signs and symptoms of fibromyalgia. Exercise will improve your muscle range of motion.

Most doctors agree that medications, injections, and therapy alone will not be able to eliminate your pain, but rather it will help you to manage your pain and cope with it better. Taking steroids to treat your fibromyalgia will not improve your symptoms of pain. People with other muscle or bone conditions such as rheumatoid arthritis do respond well to steroids. However, nonsteroidal anti-inflammatory medications such as ibuprofen may relieve or at least decrease your muscle pain.

The primary goal in treating your fibromyalgia is to attempt to break the pain cycle. One way of accomplishing this goal is to correct any disturbance in your sleep pattern. Amitriptyline (Elavil) can be an important drug in restoring your sleep. Numerous studies have shown that getting enough sleep can significantly reduce your pain. If you are allergic to amitriptyline, cyclobenzaprine (Flexeril) can be substituted. In some people, nonsteroidal anti-inflammatory medications such as ibuprofen can be successfully used. Amantadine hydrochloride (Symmetrel) also may be used. This medication is an antiviral as well as an anti-Parkinson medication. Serotonin reuptake inhibitors (Paxil) may also have a positive effect on reducing your pain. There are new two drugs approved by the FDA for the treatment of fibromyalgia; Lyrica (an anticonvulsant) and Cymbalta (an antidepressant).

Nerve stimulation is another method of relieving pain that you may find helpful. A TENS unit (Transcutaneous Electrical Nerve Stimulator) is useful in managing fibromyalgia pain in many patients. This small battery-powered instrument has two to four patches that are placed over your painful muscle areas. Electrical impulses will stimulate the nerves around your areas of pain. This stimulation will cause the production of the pain-relieving chemical enkephalin into your spinal cord. Enkephalins will diminish the intensity of your pain signals that ultimately reach your brain. Another useful device that is gaining in popularity is a muscle stimulator. This device has six to eight patches that are placed over your painful muscle areas. The muscle stimulator machine will stimulate and work your muscles until they are fatigued and weakened. It is possible for your muscles that have been weakened by the fibromyalgia to be strengthened this way.

Be aware of the "leaking gut" theory as a cause of fibromyalgia. If large proteins leak into your gastrointestinal circulation, your immune system may become overactive. You can then experience an antibody response that causes you to have generalized body pain. Some individuals that have fibromyalgia from this cause can be treated successfully with a gluten free diet, colostrums supplements or hyperimmune eggs. A psychologist can help you deal with the suffering aspect of your pain. Your psychologist also may want to teach you biofeedback. This is a good way for you to learn relaxing techniques that can significantly reduce your pain. Your psychologist may want you to listen to a CD or cassette tapes at home. Aromatherapy also could be effective for helping you manage your pain. This method is more effective in women because their scent perception is better than a man's. You may also find that hypnosis can decrease your pain intensity as well. You may want to try self-hypnosis as another modality for the management of your chronic pain.

Insomina is common in fibromyalgia. Chronic insomnia alone impacts 10% to 15% of adults. Epidemiologic data indicate that pain, fatigue, and mood disturbance are common correlates of persistent insomnia. Your physician must try to correct your insomnia. A good night's rest increases norepinerpherine and serotonin in your central nervous system. These are two biochemicals in your body that can decrease your pain. Fibromyalgia is associated with insomnia. The same is true for RSD/CRPS. Significant sleep disturbances are reported by 80% of patients with CRPS. RSD/CRPS and fibromyalgia patients have severe influences on the quality of life in these patients. Fibromyalgia is associated with significant depression. Complex regional pain syndrome like fibromyalgia is a severe disabling pain disorder that results in physical as well as emotional (depression)and financial consequences to patients.

Patients with a fibromyalgia syndrome can present with myofascial trigger points just like RSD/CRPS. Just like RSD/CRPS, fibromyalgia patients may have autonomic phenomena like skin reddening and sweating. Younger female (37 years) fibromyalgia patients presenting with autonomic phenomena should be examined for a myofascial pain syndromes as well. Substance P, a pain transmitter is elevated in patients suffering from fibromyalgia. A hypotheses exists that the distal tibial fracture model of a rat simulates RSD/CRPS. Leg immobilization alone can generate a syndrome resembling RSD/CRPS, and substance P contributes to the vascular and pain changes observed in these models. Substance P induced plasma protein extravasations are increased in RSD/CRPS patients on both the affected and unaffected limbs. The underlying mechanism might be impaired substance P inactivation. These findings further support the hypothesis that neurogenic inflammation plays an important role in the initiation of RSD/CRPS and possibly fibromyalgia.

Sometimes fibromyalgia can be confused with RSD/CRPS. You need to be aware that RSD/CRPS can spread from the injured area to the other extremities in your body. If your RSD/CRPS is confined to your arm or leg, the diagnosis of CRPS is much easier than RSD/CRPS that has spread to your other three extremities. RSD/CRPS is then very difficult to distinguish from fibromyalgia. For example, if you have RSD/CRPS of your hand, it can spread to the rest of your extremities. Therefore, it is necessary for you to have a basic understanding of fibromyalgia. While occasionally someone afflicted with fibromyalgia is told that he or she may have Reflex Sympathetic Dystrophy (RSD/CRPS), it is not uncommon for someone with RSD/CRPS to be told he has fibromyalgia. Unfortunately, this only adds confusion to those with either of these disorders.

The hallmark of RSD/CRPS is cold sensitivity in the presence of blood vessel instability and significant sweating in the affected extremity in addition to an abnormal skin color (usually blue or purple). Symptoms usually begin after an identifiable, causative event. It has been shown that barometric changes can sensitize pain fibers. As a result of this increased sensation, your pain can significantly increase. In patients with RSD/CRPS, the weather-sensitive component may manifest itself as pain that increases with barometric changes. This is a noticeable worsening and a major feature in those with RSD/CRPS. In contrast, Fibromyalgia patients may also have weather sensitivity; however, this problem is not a hallmark feature of the disorder. Fibromyalgia patients tend to have more generalized pain, earlier complaints of fatigue, and a history of immune system over-activity or persistent infection when compared to the RSD/CRPS patient. Fibromyalgia patients are less likely to have an inciting event that they can relate their symptoms to. Despite these variations, there may be considerable overlap between the two diagnostic groups.

For example, an RSD/CRPS patient whose symptoms seem to have spread may look very much as if they have Fibromyalgia. This is because the new areas of pain may have no obvious inciting event, are less likely to be associated with contracture or bone loss, and are often associated with increasing fatigue. While it is important to evaluate new symptoms to determine if there has been a progression of RSD/CRPS, spread can usually be proven in only a minority of cases. New symptoms may: represent an unrelated problem, provide evidence that the disease has developed into Chronic Regional Pain Syndrome (CRPS) that is independent of sympathetic pain or be a clue that there is an infection or immunologic compromise.

If the previously mentioned hallmark changes for RSD/CRPS occur, or if thermographic or bone scan findings suggest objective findings then a true spread of RSD/CRPS can be diagnosed. Likewise it should be recognized that a Fibromyalgia patient's symptoms might progressively worsen to the point that the sympathetic component becomes dominant and RSD/CRPS features develop. While this is not common, if it does happen, treatment should be aggressive. Although there can be considerable overlap between patients with sympathetic pain who do not develop full blown RSD/CRPS and fibromyalgia patients who are weather-sensitive, a skilled clinician should be able to differentiate between the two conditions in the majority of cases. What is helpful is that the treatments for both entities are similar other than spinal cord stimulators or sympathetic injections are not indicated for the treatment of fibromyalgia. In RSD/CRPS patients, muscle cramps (spasms and dystonia) can be treated with clonazepam and baclofen. Muscles stiffness may be treated with muscle relaxants such as tizanidine (Zanaflex), baclofen or clonazepam (Klonopin).

Sometimes fibromyalgia can be confused with RSD/CRPS. You need to be aware that RSD/CRPS can spread from the injured area to the other extremities in your body. For example, if you have RSD/CRPS of your hand, it can spread to the rest of your extremities. Therefore, it is necessary for you to have a basic understanding of fibromyalgia. While occasionally someone afflicted with fibromyalgia is told that he or she may have Reflex Sympathetic Dystrophy (RSD/CRPS), it is not uncommon for someone with RSD/CRPS to be told he has Fibromyalgia. Unfortunately, this only adds confusion to those with either of these disorders.

Despite these differences, there may well be considerable overlay between the two diagnostic groups. For example, an RSD/CRPS patient whose symptoms seem to have spread may appear as if he/she has fibromyalgia. This is because the new areas of pain may have no apparent provocative occurrence, are less likely to be linked with muscle contractures or bone loss, and can be associated with chronic fatigue. While it is important to evaluate new symptoms to determine if there has been a succession of RSD/CRPS, spread of RSD/CRPS can usually be verified in only a minority of cases. New symptoms in a RSD/CRPS patient may represent an unrelated problem, provide evidence that the disease has developed into chronic RSD/CRPS that is independent of sympathetic pain, or be a suspicion that there is unknown infection or immunologic compromise.

11. Myofascial Pain and RSD/CRPS

Myofascial pain syndrome is a chronic local or regional musculoskeletal pain disorder that may involve either a single muscle or a muscle group. The pain may be of a burning, stabbing, aching or nagging quality. Importantly, where the patient experiences the pain may not be where the myofascial pain generator is located. This is known as referred pain. Following the onset of CRPS, a patient may demonstrate myofascial trigger points. You can develop a severe myofascial pain syndrome with reflex sympathetic dystrophy. If trigger points are present, treatment should consist of specific myofascial trigger point therapy, beginning with desensitization and gentle massage on the trigger points. Allodynia can be reduced and further physical therapy used to decrease the myofascial muscle pain. Trigger point injections may subsequently be effective for resolution of the extremity pain.

Almost everyone has experienced muscle pain a sometime. You may have had muscle pain if you were active playing sports or working in your garden. A myofascial pain syndrome is a soft tissue disorder of your muscles that can cause you not only to have pain for a long time, but it can also cause you to on occasion, have some disability. Your overall activities of daily living, including work, recreation and social interaction can be significantly affected. Myofascial pain is pain related to muscle injury or overuse resulting in taut bands and palpable areas of pain that is referred to other muscular areas of your body. Injury to you rm or leg can result in myofascial pain. RSD is frequently caused by an injury to your arm or leg. The pain can be dull, sharp or burning. You may suffer from sleep deprivation depression and anxiety like fibromyalgia. Your doctor may make a diagnosis of myofascial pain if you cry out or wince and withdraw away from light palpation on an area of your body

Muscle strains and ligament sprains can cause pain in your muscles and can contribute to the onset of a myofascial pain syndrome. The pain intensity of myofascial disorders can vary from painless decreases in range of motion about your arms, legs, neck, and lower back, which are common in older individuals, to pain that is agonizing and incapacitating. This latter type of pain is seen if you are young and are extremely active.

Acute myofascial pain can decrease your activities of daily living. If it becomes chronic, it can be a major cause of time lost at work. The good news is that most myofascial pain can be relieved with an appropriate diagnosis and specific treatment. Pressing on the tender spots on your body can identify myofascial trigger points. When you tender area is pressed, you will have pain in other areas of your body that are away from the area being examined. Fibromyalgia pain does not cause referred pain when tender areas are palpated. The pains in the other areas are referred pain patterns that demonstrate trigger points. Myofascial trigger points occur when there is trauma to your muscle or prolonged tension on your muscle from slouching over a desk or slouching over a worktable. This slouching results in disruption of your muscle cells.

When your muscle cell becomes disrupted, your cells release calcium. Calcium released inside of your muscle cell stimulates more contractions of your muscle. A prolonged contraction will exceed the available oxygen, glucose, and other nutrients that are needed for the energy to allow your muscle to continue to contract. With a sustained contraction, you run out of oxygen as well as other nutrients. This allows your muscle cell to build up a substance called lactic acid which stimulates muscle pain fibers.

Substances that cause your body to produce pain-causing substances are prostaglandins that sensitize pain fibers or substance P (a pain neuro-transmitter) that is involved in pain transmission. These pain transmitters then stimulate nerve endings around your muscle cells. These nerve endings go to other structures in your body. This is why you notice a referred pain pattern when you have a myofascial pain syndrome. You will notice nodular, ropelike bands under your painful muscles when you have myofascial pain syndrome. The lack of oxygen in your muscle tissue will cause some of your muscle cells to die. This will cause scar tissue to form about your muscles. This scar tissue gives you the nodular feeling when you press over these painful areas.

Not all pain in your muscles is from myofascial pain. Sometimes arthritis can cause muscle pain surrounding your joints. Myopathy is a disease of muscles that can occur and cause you to have muscle pain. If you have a disc herniation, you can have referred pain to your muscles as well. Rocky Mountain Spotted Fever or Lyme disease can also cause you to have muscle pain. A myofascial trigger point in your muscle needs to be distinguished from tender areas around your ligaments as well as around your bone. The diagnosis of your myofascial pain syndrome is made by your health-care provider's history and physical examination and expertise. No laboratory tests are useful for the diagnosis of this syndrome. If you have the myofascial pain syndrome, you will complain of localized muscle pain and tenderness as well as the referred pain. If you have myofascial trigger points around your head and neck, you may complain of headaches as well as problems with your vision. Remember that you can have myofascial trigger points in one muscle or many muscles.

To make a diagnosis of myofascial trigger points, you must have painful areas in a muscle that is noted by your doctor on physical examination. These painful areas must be nodular and must be reproducible. Different amounts of pressure from your examining health-care provider will give you referred pain. If you truly have myofascial pain your doctor will record whether you have a "jump sign" noted on physical examination. This means that when your doctor applies pressure on your trigger point, you jump away from the pressure. Your health-care provider will usually notice a twitch about the area that has pressure applied to it. At the time of your examination, your health care provided will notice that your pain diminishes with stretching or following injection of your muscle with a local anesthetic.

Your trigger points are classified as either active or latent. Active trigger points occur following acute muscle trauma. The latent trigger point on the other hand does not cause you to have pain at rest but can cause you to have restriction of movement about a certain part of your body. Latent trigger points are from a previous muscle injury. A latent trigger point can persist for years after recovery from an injury. Latent trigger points can predispose you to have pain with overuse of your previously injured muscle. Sometimes in cold weather, your muscle will contract and cause you to have pain. Remember, only the active trigger points cause pain. The latent trigger points cause pain when they become active. Normal muscles do not have trigger points that can be felt or have areas that can cause you pain when touched. You should feel your normal muscles. Normal muscles do not have ropelike, nodular areas or tender areas to pressure and exhibit no observable twitch when your health-care provider palpates your muscle. Furthermore, you will not have referred pain with this applied pressure.

You can have different degrees of severity of myofascial pain. Some trigger points are much more sensitive than others. An extremely sensitive trigger point can cause you to have greater referred nerve pain than a less-severe or intense trigger point. Myofascial pain is usually not symmetrical on either side of your body. However, medical conditions that cause muscle pain such as fibromyalgia are symmetrical. Trigger points are usually activated by overuse of muscles. You can stretch your muscle beyond its normal capability, which will cause your muscle to become injured. Bleeding can occur within your muscle following injury, which may cause scar formation in your muscle.

Active trigger points can develop in your muscles following excessive, repetitive, or sustained motions. For example, if you work in a warehouse and load heavy boxes all day over months, you can begin to develop active trigger points. Common areas of trigger point pain include your neck, arms, shoulders, face, back and legs. Emotional stress can also cause trigger points. Stress can cause your muscles to stay in a contracted state. When your muscles are contracted for a length of time as previously stated, you lose oxygen and other nutrients to your muscle tissues. You must attempt to relax and do breathing exercises and range-of-motion exercises to decrease your pain. Heat and cold my help decrease your pain. Myofascial pain can vary in pain severity from hour by hour or from day by day. The stress required to produce pain is variable. Again, if you are under much stress, it does not take much additional muscle stress to produce myofascial pain.

The amount of stress that is needed to make your latent trigger point become an active trigger point depends on your degree of conditioning of your muscles and your exercise tolerance as well. If you do not exercise and do aerobic activity and are under a lot of stress, you have susceptibility to develop active painful trigger points. If your muscles are stiff, you should avoid placing cold packs on a muscle that may already be contracted. You should use heat instead of the cold. Viral illnesses can also cause muscle pain. If you have a virus, do not put cold packs on your muscles. A virus will activate chemicals in your body that activate pain signals. That is why you ache all over your body when you have the flu. With a viral infection, you can have pain in all of your joints as well as headaches and muscle pain.

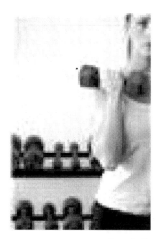

Figure 1. A muscle injury can cause myofascial pain. This pain can be superimposed with RSD/CRPS. Trigger point injections can be helpful in the injured muscle.

Myofascial pain may outlast any precipitating traumatic musculoskeletal event. The pain duration is of myofascial pain is longer in duration than the muscle strain duration. The duration depends on your overall muscular prior to an injury. If you are a professional football player for example, you can have a muscle strain and never develop trigger points. If you are not physically fit, a minor muscle strain can result in myfascial pain. A problem occurs when you are injured; your muscles have developed a way of trying to prevent further pain. In doing so, these other muscles will cause your injured muscle to be protected. Eventually your active trigger points will become latent.

If you rest your muscle and use a splint or an elastic bandage, your active trigger point may revert to become a latent trigger point. Occasionally you may do an activity that will activate your latent trigger point. This not unusual and you should expect this occurrence on occasion. Many of your muscles around your active trigger point can decrease their function, causing your muscles to become weak. If enough of your muscles lose a significant portion of their function, you can develop weakness of an entire extremity.

Myofascial pain is caused by pressure over your muscles. When you are lying in bed, you may have some pressure on your body in the area of the trigger points from your mattress. This pressure from your bed can cause you to have pain. On the other hand, be aware that sleep disturbances can cause your muscles to contract and become stiff and can worsen your myofascial pain syndrome. If your health-care provider does not visually notice spasms of your painful muscle, this individual may snap your muscle to see if you truly have a myofascial trigger point. This essentially amounts to pinching and pulling your muscle up. When this happens, usually your muscle will demonstrate a visible muscle twitch demonstrating a myofascial trigger point. This muscle response can also be seen if you have latent trigger points. The highest incidence of the onset of trigger points occurs between ages 31 and 50. When you are over 50, maximum activity could cause you to suffer from myofascial pain. As you continue to age and reduce your activity as a result of pain, your range of motion as a result of latent trigger points will become manifest. Many health-care providers are aware of myofascial trigger points.

Chiropractors treat myofascial trigger points, as do physical therapists. Acupuncturists, anesthesiologists, dentists, pediatricians, rheumatologists, and specialists in physical medicine and rehabilitation all treat myofascial pain syndrome. The manner in which each of these health-care providers treats myofascial pain will vary from each of the health-care provider specialties. If your pain is not relieved with conservative measures another method that can decrease your pain is a botulism toxin injection into your painful muscles. This drug is a gram-negative bacterium. In small doses it can relax or even paralyze small muscle fibers. The relief from the injection of the Botox can last up to three months. The problem with the Botox injection is that some individuals develop what appears to be fever and generalized joint pain associated with the bacteria that gets into their bloodstream. These side effects should however, subside over several days.

Prevention of myofascial trigger points should be considered. This may be accomplished by doing stretching exercises both before and immediately after engaging in strenuous exercise. This concept may also be used if you are not physically fit and want to work in your garden for example. Do stretching exercises both before and after gardening. This may prevent the onset of myofascial pain. The pathophysiology of myofascial pain remains somewhat of a mystery due to limited clinical research; however, based on case reports and medical observation, investigators think it may develop from a muscle lesion or excessive strain on a particular muscle or muscle group, ligament or tendon. It is thought that the lesion or the strain prompts the development of a "trigger point" that, in turn, causes pain.

In addition to the local or regional pain, people with a myofascial pain syndrome also can suffer from depression, fatigue and behavioral disturbances, as with all chronic pain conditions. Recognition of this syndrome is difficult and requires the physician to have a precise understanding of the body's anatomy. Trigger points can be identified by pain produced upon digital palpation. In diagnosing myofascial pain syndrome, two types of trigger points can be distinguished:

1. Active trigger point; an area of exquisite tenderness that is usually located in a skeletal muscle and is associated with local or regional pain.

2. latent trigger point; a dormant area that can potentially behave like an active trigger point.

The best treatments for myofascial pain syndrome are active and passive physical therapy methods. There is also the "stretch and spray" technique, in which the muscle with the trigger point is sprayed along its length with a coolant such as fluorimethane, and then stretched slowly. Trigger point injection, whereby local anesthesia is injected directly into the trigger point, also is used. At times, corticosteroids and botulinum toxin can be injected. Massage therapy also can be of significant benefit in some patients. Often a combination of physical therapy, trigger point injections and massage are needed in refractory chronic cases.

CRPS can be associated with myofascial trigger points. Sudden trauma to musculoskeletal tissues like muscles, ligaments, tendons, and bursae. Lack of range of motion can cause extremity myofascial pain. The fascia is a connective tissue which spreads throughout the body from a patient's head to foot. The fascia surrounds muscles, bones, nerves, blood vessels and organs of the body. The fascia itself contains many pain fibers. You need to be aware that on occasion, trigger points can produce autonomic nervous system changes such as flushing of the skin, hypersensitivity of areas of the skin, or sweating in areas. These symptoms are similar to those of CRPS. An active trigger point when treated will become quiet. If an injury that causes CRPS occurs, the quiet trigger points can become active. Sometimes addressing treatment of the trigger points will resolve the CRPS.

12. Anticonvulsant Medications

RSD/CRPS is a chronic neuropathic pain syndrome. It causes nerve pain. One pharmacologic treatment of RSD/CRPS pain is utilization of an anticonvulsant medication. Anticonvulsant drugs have been used for the management of neuropathic (damaged nerve) pain since the 1960s. These drugs interfere with the total number of pain signals that travel to your brain. This type of drug seems to be especially effective for managing sharp, shooting and lancinating pain. It is possible that anticonvulsants stabilize excitable nerve membranes, limit neuronal hyperexcitability, and inhibit transynaptic neuronal impulses in the CNS. Gabapentin (neurontin), a GABA-mimetic, seems currently (since 1994) to be the anticonvulsant used most widely in North America in the treatment of CRPS/RSD. Lyrica (pregabilin is however becoming very popular).

Gabapentin binds in the outer layer of the neocortex (outer layer of your brain) of your brain and the hippocampus. At one time it was thought that gabapentin's anticonvulsant effects may be mediated by increasing the promoted release of GABA. When GABA is released in your spinal cord, pain signals going toward your brain are decreased. It has both analgesic and antianxiety effects. In the formalin test with mice, gabapentin selectively blocks nociception associated with inflammation, suggesting a central site of action, perhaps by blocking the sensitization of dorsal horn neurones that occurs during inflammation. It is now known that gabapentin and Lyrica act on voltage sensitive alpha 2 delta receptors to decrease pain. Gabapentin appears to differ from the other anticonvulsants in its mechanism of action. Gabapentin is not metabolized by the liver and can therefore safely be given with other anticonvulsants. It is well tolerated and has few adverse effects (mostly drowziness, fatigue and dizziness). These side effects these tend to decrease with continued usage. Other anticonvulsants used for RSD are phenytoin (Dilantin), carbamezapine (Tegretol) and valproic acid (Depakot).

The clinical impression of these drugs is that they are useful for chronic neuropathic (nerve damage) pain, especially when the pain is lancinating or burning. Remember that RSD pain is burning. Pain is usually the natural consequence of tissue injury resulting in approximately forty million medical appointments per year. In general, following most injuries, as the healing process commences, the pain and tenderness associated with your injury will resolve. Unfortunately, some individuals experience pain without an obvious injury or suffer pain that persists for months or years after their initial injury. This pain condition is neuropathic in nature and accounts for a large number of patients presenting to pain clinics with chronic pain.

Following any tissue injury (nerve, muscle, bone, etc) your nervous system sounds an alarm to your brain to make you aware that you have been injured. Rather than your nervous system functioning properly to sound an alarm regarding tissue injury, in neuropathic pain, the peripheral or central nervous systems are malfunctioning and become the cause of the pain. In other words, after your nerve has healed it may still transmit pain signals. An example is a car alarm. The alarm will sound if your vehicle is being tampered with. This is normal. Now imagine that your alarm sounds when no one is near your car. Somehow there is a short circuit. The same occurs within your nervous system.

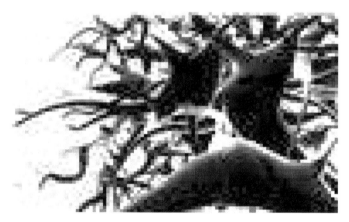

Figure 1. Neurons are intertwined in your nervous system. Pain signals are transmitted between gaps between your axons and dendrites. Anticonvulsant medications can interrupt pain signals by blocking transmission of these pain signals.

Neuropathic pain is a complex, pain state that usually is accompanied by nerve injury. With neuropathic pain, the nerve fibers themselves may be damaged, dysfunctional or injured. These damaged nerve fibers send incorrect signals to other pain centers. The impact of nerve injury includes a change in nerve function both at the site of injury and areas around the injury. Symptoms may include: shooting and burning pain and tingling and numbness. In order to understand the effects of antiseizure drugs, you need to be aware that these drugs can block the ion (calcium and sodium) channels that are present throughout your nervous system. Ion channels are pore-forming proteins that help to establish and control a small electrical gradient between the inside and outside of your nerve cells. When ions flow in and out of your neuron, this electrical gradient ceases and pain signals subsequently cease to be transmitted to your brain. Calcium and sodium channed anticonvulsant drugs block the pores or channels. When these drugs drop off of these channels, you will experience pain again.

Antiseizure drugs are frequently used in pain management. It is not known exactly how anticonvulsants work to reduce pain. They may block the flow of pain signals from your brain and spinal cord. Some anticonvulsant drugs may work better than others for certain conditions. Neuropathic pain, is a form of chronic pain caused by an injury to or a disease of your peripheral or central nervous system. It does not respond well to traditional pain therapies like opioids or nonsteroidal anti-inflammatory drugs.

In neuropathic pain, it has shown that a number of pathophysiological and biochemical changes take place in your nervous system as a result of an insult to a nerve. This property of the nervous system to adapt to external stimuli plays a crucial role in the onset and maintenance of pain symptoms. Carbamazepine (Tegretol), the first anticonvulsant studied in clinical trials, probably alleviates pain by decreasing conductance in sodium channels and inhibits ectopic nerve discharges. Results from clinical trials have been positive in the treatment of trigeminal neuralgia, painful diabetic neuropathy and postherpetic neuralgia with this medication.

Gabapentin (Neurontin) and pregabilin (Lyrica) have the most clearly demonstrated analgesic effects for the treatment of neuropathic pain, specifically for the treatment of painful diabetic neuropathy and postherpetic neuralgia. Based on the positive results of these studies and its favorable adverse effect profile, gabapentin or pregabilin should be considered the first choice of therapy for neuropathic pain. Evidence for the efficacy of phenytoin as an antinociceptive agent is, at best, weak to modest. Lamotrigine (Lamictal) on the other hand has good potential to modulate and control neuropathic pain.

There is a potential for phenobarbital, clonazepam, valproic acid, topiramate, pregabalin and tiagabine to have antihyperalgesic and antinociceptive activities based on result in animal models of neuropathic pain, but the efficacy of these drugs in the treatment of human neuropathic pain has not yet been fully determined in clinical trials. The role of anticonvulsant drugs in the treatment of neuropathic pain is evolving and has been clearly demonstrated with gabapentin and carbamazepine. Further advances in our understanding of the mechanisms underlying neuropathic pain syndromes and well-designed clinical trials should further the opportunities to establish the role of anticonvulsants in the treatment of neuropathic pain.

If you have had a direct injury to one of your nerves, you may benefit from an anticonvulsant drug. The clinical impression is that these drugs are useful for the treatment of chronic neuropathic pain, especially when the pain is lancinating or burning. There are seven drugs that are useful in neuropathic (nerve injury) pain; pregabilin (Lyrica), gabapentin (Neurontin), carbamazipine (Tegretol), valproic acid (Depakote), clonazepamm (Klonopin), phenytoin (Dilantin) ,zonisamide (Zonegran)) and lamotrigine (Lamictal). Neurontin is an effective drug for the treatment of neuropathic pain but Lyrica is becoming widely used as previously mentioned in the management of many pain syndromes. It has fewer side effects than other anticonvulsant drugs. These drugs can be useful for the treatment of shingles, diabetic neuropathy and fibromyalgia. Reflex Sympathetic Dystrophy, diabetic neuropathy migraine headaches, sciatica, radiculitis, and pain associated with multiple sclerosis may respond to either of these drugs.

If you experience sharp shooting pain, these drugs may be helpful in decreasing your pain. If you experience side effects from either drug, other anticonvulsant medications are available. Oxcarbazepine (Trileptal), lamotrigine (Lamictal), topiramate (Topamax), and zonisamide (Zonegran) may also be effective in reducing pain caused by diabetic neuropathy and postherpetic neuralgia. Lyrica is now FDA approved in 2007 for the treatment of fibromyalgia. Anticonvulsant drugs are effective in the treatment of chronic neuropathic pain but were not initially thought to be useful in the management of postoperative pain. However, similar to any nerve injury, surgical tissue injury is known to produce neuroplastic changes leading to spinal sensitization and the expression of nerve in- duced pain. Gabapentin (Neurontin) may decrease post surgical pain. The pharmacological effects of anticonvulsant drugs, which may be important in the modulation of these postoperative neural changes, include suppres- sion of sodium channel, calcium channel and glutamate receptor activity at peripheral, spinal and supraspinal sites.

Your doctor may obtain a complete blood count and liver tests before prescribing some of these anticonvulsant drugs (e.g. Tegretol). Your doctor will give you a 4 to 6 week trial of the drug. It may take the medication this length of time to exert its effects. Therefore, if you have no pain relief after several days you should not stop the drug that was prescribed to you. Because it takes your body time to adjust to one of these medications, your doctor must adhere to the phrase "begin low and proceed slow" which means that you should be prescribed a low dose and this dose may be increased gradually over days to weeks. Anticonvulsant drugs are effective in the treatment of chronic pain but may also be useful for pain management following surgery.

Similar to any nerve injury, surgical tissue injury is known to produce tissue changes leading to spinal cord sensitization which can cause you to have pain after surgery. Gabapentin has been shown to decrease post surgery pain. Pregabilin is effective for the treatment of diabetic neuropa- thy and shingles. Pregabilin binds to calcium channels of nerves, which results in a reduction of your pain. Some health insurance plans do not pay for Lyrica because it is new and relatively expensive. However, it has been shown to be more cost effective than gabapentin. In other words, it is more effective than gabapentin for RSD/CRPS pain control. However, this drug can cause dizziness, blurred vision, drowsiness, weight gain and swelling of your legs. This medication may decrease your platelet count as well.

Some anticonvulsant medicines can cause a decrease in your platelets which can interfere with your ability to form a blood clot. If your platelets are too low, you will bruise easily. Gabapentin is effective for the man- agement of oral phantom pain following a tooth extraction. Gabapentin binds to nerve calcium channels. Gabapentin has a mild effect on pain in RSD/CRPS. It can significantly reduce a sensory deficit in the affected limb. A subpopulation of RSD/CRPS patients may therefore, benefit from gabapentin. Gabapentin is useful for the management of RSD/CRPS pain as well as facial RSD. The drug is useful in most nerve injury pain disorders. An average dose is 300 mg taken three times a day. A rare side effect has been reported with gabapentin use. A 35-year-old woman suffered a traumatic injury to her right sciatic nerve. She developed a complex regional pain syndrome and was treated with gabapentin for pain control. Three months after the initiation of gabapentin therapy (1800 mg/day), the patient reported complete cessation of her menses. The patient was weaned off the gabapentin over 6 days with return of her menses 2 weeks later. It was conclude that gabapentin has the potential to cause amenorrhea with return of menses occurring after discontinuation of the drug.

Tegretol is a drug that is chemically related to amitriptyline. It prevents repetitive discharges of your nerves. This medication works on sodium channels in your painful nerves. Inhibition of these sodium channels can decrease your pain sensations. An average dose is 200 mg every day. Side effects include dizziness, drowsiness, blurred vision and nausea. This medication can cause various forms of anemia and liver damage. As a result, your doctor will obtain a blood count and liver tests. Tegretol is rarely used today for RSD pain because of the side effects associated with this drug. Tegretol has been shown to be effective for the treatment of trigeminal neuralgia (facial pain). Some physicians use this drug for RSD pain. Depakote is given in a dose of 250 mg twice a day. This medication can cause you to have liver failure. Your doctor will monitor your liver function closely. This medicine is used when the other anti convulsant medications have been tried but failed to provide pain relief. Side effects of this drug include nausea, vomiting loss of appetite and diarrhea. Tremors and sedation may also be associated with this medication.

Klonopin may be useful for the treatment of pain associated with the burning mouth syndrome. Klonipin is useful also for the treatment of lancinating pain associated with the phantom limb syndrome. The drug may also be useful for migraine headache prophylaxis and for the treatment of trigeminal neuralgia (facial pain). The usual dose is 1 mg per day. Side effects include mood disturbances and delirium. Lethargy and sedation may also be seen. This drug has a significant sedative effect. It should be initially only taken at bedtime. It is prescribed by some neurologists for RSD/CRPS pain.

Dilantin alters sodium, calcium and potassium channels in your nerves. An average dose is 300 mg three times a day. The number of side effects associated with this drug is significant. Liver damage can occur and the drug can decrease your folic acid level in your bloodstream. A decrease in your folic acid blood level may actually cause your nerves in your arms and legs to have burning sensations.

Zonegran 's mechanisms of action suggest that it could be effective in controlling neuropathic pain symptoms. It can be effective in the management of RSD/CRPS pain. It also decreases sodium channel activity on the sodium channels of your nerves. Side effects can include a decrease in your blood sodium levels, kidney stones, visual difficulties and secondary angle-closure glaucoma. A typical dose of this medication is 300 mg per day. Side effects related to this drug include agitation, anxiety, ataxia, confusion, depression, difficulty concentrating, headache, difficulty sleeping, memory problems, stomach pain as well as liver pathology. This medication may also cause weight loss. A dry mouth and flu like syndrome may also be associated with this drug.

Lamictal also exerts its effects on sodium channels. This drug decreases the release of some pain-causing chemical from the ends of your nerves. The reason why you develop chronic pain after having acute nerve injury pain remains unclear. However, it is believed that Lamictal in addition to some of the other drugs mentioned may prevent this transformation. A typical dose will be 200 mg twice a day after starting at a low dose and going to 200 mg slowly. Adverse effects related to this drug include headaches, dizziness, blurred vision and nausea and vomiting. This medication may be of benefit for the treatment of pain associated with Reflex Sympathetic Dystrophy. Lamictal also can be effective for many kinds of neuropathic pain including that which comes from RSD/CRPS, AIDS and central brain pain as a result of a stroke. Lamictal is a seizure medicine that acts as a sodium channel blocker as previously mentioned but may exhibit some calcium channel blockade. In one study with patients who had severe refractory neuropathic pain who had failed at least two other treatments, there was an average 70% decrease in pain in 14 of 21 patients.

In early studies where lower doses of 200 mg a day or less were used, the effects were marginal. Doses of 200 to 400 mg a day divided through the day are more effective for some kinds of pain. Start The most troublesome side effect is a rare rash (called Stevens-Johnson Syndrome), which can be fatal. If you develop a rash, stop the medication immediately and notify your physician. A non-protein extract isolated from the inflamed skin of rabbits inoculated with vaccinia virus (Neurotropin, NTP) is under investigation in Japan and may be of benefit in the future for patients suffering from RSD/CRPS.

In summary, chronic pain, whether arising from nerve or any other tissue or structure, is, more often than commonly thought, the result of a mixture of pain mechanisms, and therefore there is no simple formula available to manage chronic complex pain states. The analgesic recommendations for difficult-to-treat pain syndromes include gabapentin or pregabalin in addition to an opioid or antidepressant. Topical therapies for cutaneous allodynia/hyperalgesia may be used in addition to anticonvulsant drugs. Anti-inflammatory drugs (corticosteroids for acute inflammatory neuropathic pain), IV bisphosphonates for CRPS/RSD. If sympathetic maintained pain is present.

Some medications are not anticonvulsants but act on nerves in your sympathetic nervous system. A physician may consider topical clonidine. This medicine decreases production of biochemicals that sensitize your nerves to cause sweating, swelling, discoloration and pain. A lidocaine 5% patch, may also be considered for a variety of pain states and features. The major rationale for introducing adjuvants is to better balance the efficacy and adverse effects of single drugs. The following scenarios should prompt the use of adjuvants in clinical practice: The toxic limit of a primary analgesic has been reached. The therapeutic benefit of a primary analgesic has plateaued. The primary analgesic is contraindicated because of substance abuse, aberrant behavior, organ failure, allergy, etc. An aversion to addiction and drug diversion remains a potent force that shapes physician prescribing profiles.

Patients often convey that different medications will impart distinct analgesic benefits. The presence of disabling nonpainful complaints and the need to manage symptoms such as insomnia, depression, anxiety, and fatigue that all cause worsening of the patient's quality of life and function need to be addressed by physicians.

13. Muscle Relaxants

Muscle cramps (spasms and dystonia) associated with RSD/CRPS can be treated with clonazepam and baclofen as well as with other muscle relaxants. Antispasmodics, also called muscle relaxants, are helpful in treating the symptoms of RSD/CRPS. Many patients with RSD/CRPS experience muscle spasms which aggravate the pain. Medications such as benzodiazepine, clonazepam and Zanaflex are prescribed to alleviate these spasms and aid in pain control. Muscle relaxants are effective for short-term symptomatic relief in patients with acute and chronic low back pain as well as those patients suffering from RSD/CRPS. Remember, that in an earlier chapter on myofascial pain and RSD/CRPS, that myofascial pain is not uncommon. Baclofen, a muscle relaxant may help with muscle spasms associated with RSD/CRPS in some cases. However, the incidence of drowsiness, dizziness and other side effects is high. Muscle relaxants must be used with caution. Muscle relaxants are a useful adjunct in the treatment of patients with chronic and persistent pain. There are a number of categories in muscle relaxants, but one may broadly divide them into centrally acting muscle relaxants and peripherally acting muscle relaxants.

Central mechanisms of action include activity on the glycine receptors, as seen with the muscle relaxant properties of benzodiazepines, or on the GABA receptors, as seen with benzodiazepines and baclofen. Baclofen has been used to treat the spasticity of multiple sclerosis; it may also be used to treat muscle spasm associated with radiculopathy. Cyclobenzaprine differs from amitriptyline by two hydrogen ions, and it retains many of the side effects of amitriptyline (e.g., dry mouth, constipation, irregular heartbeats). Muscle relaxants are effective for short-term symptomatic relief in patients with acute and chronic low back pain as well as with some RSD/CRPS pain. However, the incidence of drowsiness, dizziness and other side effects is high. Muscle relaxants must be used with caution. Muscle relaxants are a useful adjunct in the treatment of patients with chronic and persistent pain. There are a number of categories in muscle relaxants, but one may broadly divide them into (1) centrally acting muscle relaxants and (2) peripherally acting muscle relaxants.

If your muscles are tense, you can have decreased oxygen in your muscle tissue that can cause you to experience pain. Muscle relaxants are drugs that decrease tension in your muscles. These drugs can be useful in pain management. Muscle relaxants are not really a single class of drugs, but are a group of different drugs and each of these drugs can have an overall sedative effect on your body. These drugs other than dantrolene do not act directly on your muscles, but they act in your brain and are more of a total body relaxant.

Skeletal muscle relaxants are drugs that relax striated muscles (those that control your skeleton). Skeletal muscle relaxants may be used for relief of spasticity in neuromuscular diseases, such as multiple sclerosis, as well as for spinal cord injury and stroke. They may also be used for pain relief in minor strain injuries and control of the muscle symptoms of tetanus. The muscle relaxants may be divided into only two groups, centrally acting and peripherally acting. The centrally acting group, which appears to act on the central nervous system, while only dantrolene has a direct action at the level of the nerve-muscle connection.

Dantrolene (Dantrium) has been used to prevent or treat malignant hyperthermia (severe elevation of your body temperature and muscle contractions during anesthesia) in surgery. When your muscles are tense, blood flow in your muscles can decrease. The decreased blood flow decreases your muscle oxygen level that can cause you to experience pain just as if your heart muscle has decreased oxygen following a heart attack. Decreased oxygen to your heart muscle is the reason you experience angina.

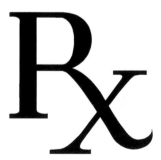

Your doctor must be aware of drug interactions and side effects when prescribing muscle relaxants.

Strains, sprains, and other muscle and joint injuries that may occur in RSD/CRPS patients can result in pain, stiffness, and muscle spasms. Muscle relaxants do not heal the injuries, but they do relax muscles and help ease discomfort. Muscle relaxants exert their effects by acting on the central nervous system. In the United States, they are available only with a physician's prescription. Several examples include; carisoprodol (Soma), cyclobenzaprine (Flexeril), and methocarbamol (Robaxin).

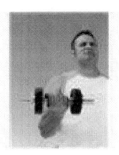

Figure 1. Muscle relaxants may help relieve muscle pains.

Most drugs come only in pill form. However, methocarbamol (Robaxin) is available in both tablet and injectable forms. Muscle relaxants are usually prescribed along with rest, exercise, physical therapy, or other treatments. One muscle relaxant, Zanaflex (tizanidine) does provide pain relief by decreasing Substance P which is one of your body's pain signal transmitters. Substance P has been implicated in RSD/CRPS pain. This medication is also helpful in decreasing pain associated with fibromyalgia. Although the muscle relaxant drugs may provide you with pain relief, they should never be considered a substitute for other forms of treatment like physical therapy. Because muscle relaxants exert their effects on your central nervous system, they may potentate the effects of alcohol and other drugs. They may also add to the effects of anesthetics, including those used for dental procedures. For this reason, anyone who takes these drugs should not drive; operate machinery, or any activity that might be dangerous.

People with certain medical conditions or who are taking certain other medicines can have problems if they take muscle relaxants. Diabetics should be aware that metaxalone (Skelaxin) may cause false test results on one type of test that detects sugar in your urine. Patients with epilepsy should be cautioned that taking the muscle relaxant methocarbamol might increase the likelihood of seizures.

Common side effects of muscle relaxants are visual changes, such as double vision or blurred vision; dizziness; lightheadedness; drowsiness; and dry mouth. These problems usually go away as your body adjusts to the drug and do not require medical treatment. Methocarbamol and chlorzoxazone may cause temporary color changes in your urine. Other side effects are stomach cramps, nausea and vomiting, constipation, diarrhea, hiccups, clumsiness or unsteadiness, confusion, nervousness, restlessness, irritability, flushed or red face, headache, heartburn, weakness, trembling, and sleep problems. More serious side effects are not common, but may occur. Anyone who experiences breathing problems, facial swelling, fainting, unusually fast or unusually slow heartbeat, fever, tightness in the chest, rash, itching, hives, burning, stinging, red, or bloodshot eyes, or unusual thoughts or dreams after taking muscle relaxants should seek medical help promptly. Parafon Forte can cause liver pathology (injury) in some individuals. The reaction is rare, but you can develop the following symptoms: fever, rash, loss of appetite, nausea, vomiting, fatigue, pain in the upper right part of the abdomen, dark urine, or yellow skin or eyes.

Muscle relaxants may interact with some other medicines. The effects of a drug may either be lessened or potentiated. When this occurs, the effects of one or both of the drugs may change or the risk of side effects may be greater with either drug. Anyone taking muscle relaxants should let their physician know all other medicines, including over-the-counter or nonprescription medicines that he or she is taking. Some patients for example, receive muscle relaxants from an emergency department. They may not tell their treating physician. If they develop side effects, the primary care physician would not know what is causing any new symptoms. Most muscle relaxants are centrally acting. Central mechanisms of action include activity on the glycine receptors, as seen with the muscle relaxant properties of benzodiazepines, or on the GABA receptors, as seen with benzodiazepines and baclofen. Baclofen has been used to treat the spasticity of multiple sclerosis; it may also be used to treat muscle spasm associated with radiculopathy and RSD/CRPS.

This indication is not approved by the Food and Drug Administration (FDA) because the primary activity for this drug has been for myelopathies (muscle injuries). Metaxalone has a role, as do other muscle relaxants, such as carisoprodol and methocarbamol. Cyclobenzaprine

(Flexeril) has atropine-like side effects. Cyclobenzaprine differs from amitriptyline by two hydrogen ions, and it retains many of the side effects of amitriptyline (e.g., dry mouth, constipation, irregular heartbeats.

Some of these muscle relaxant drugs are antispasticity medications used to treat muscle spasms and are usually associated with disorders of your nervous system. A muscle spasm is an involuntary increase in your muscle tone that that occurs when you stretch your muscle. The cause of the spasm is not known but may be related to a decrease in your body's nervous system's ability to be able to control muscle contractions. Drugs that decrease spasms are called antispasmodic drugs and include drugs like Valium (benzodiazepine), baclofen (Lioresal), Zanaflex (tizanidine) or dantrolene. Each of these drugs can exert their effects for a long time. Shorter acting medications will be described below.

Botulism toxin administered into your muscle can decrease pain from muscle spasms or muscle dysfunction. These toxins (7 total A-G) prevent release of a chemical called acetylcholine from the nerve ending that goes to your muscle. This action can stop muscle spasms. Botulism toxins A and B are commonly used in a medical practice. These toxins can be used to manage pain associated with whiplash disorders, some headaches, torticolis and low back pain. Botulism toxin can relieve your pain for 3 months.It can take two weeks for the toxin to exert its effects. Botulism toxin injections can cause you to experience mild side effects. These effects may be a fever or mild joint pain.

Benzodiazepines are used for anxiety and seizure treatment, but Valium and Klonopin can both be used for muscle relaxation. Klonopin is used for the treatment of RSD/CRPS. These drugs exert their effects by acting in your spinal cord. These drugs are useful if you have a history of a spinal cord injury. These drugs can last for a long time once they have been introduced into your body. Valium should not be used long term. You should know Valium is a depressant and can worsen depression associated with chronic pain.

Baclofen is another powerful drug that works in your spinal cord. This drug is frequently used in patients with spinal cord injury or multiple sclerosis. Baclofen causes less sedation than benzodiazipines. However baclofen can cause some drowsiness. A sedative is a medicine used to treat restlessness. A pump with tubing placed into your spinal cord can administer baclofen continuously throughout your spinal fluid. Dantrolene affects the muscle spasm by direct action on the muscle itself. It is used in spinal cord injuries and for the treatment of spasms associated with cerebral palsy.

Tizanidine (Zanaflex) exerts its effects on your central nervous system. It is frequently used for the treatment of muscle spasms associated with rheumatoid arthritis. This drug also decreases substance P that is a pain neurotransmitter. Because this drug can decrease your blood pressure, you should use it with caution if you have a history of hypertension. The drugs mentioned above can have a long duration. Other drugs are available that have shorter actions. These types of drugs are used for short periods following muscle injuries. These drugs may also be used following surgery. They are not used to treat muscle spasms.

Carisoprodol (Soma) has sedative properties as well as muscle relaxant properties. This drug should be used for muscle pain. It will not however, relieve muscle spasms. This drug furthermore, may decrease your ability to fall asleep. Methocarbamol (Robaxin) is a sedative and decreases muscle pain by its sedative action. It has no muscle relaxant effects.

Cyclobenzaprine is a drug that is chemically related in structure to amitriptyline (Elavil). This drug does not act on muscles but exerts its effects on your brain. It causes sedation. However, this drug can reduce muscle pain and tenderness. Remember that all muscle relaxant drugs may cause severe sedation. You should not drive a car or operate machinery when taking muscle relaxants.

Baclofen, when administered into your spinal fluid, may cause severe central nervous system (CNS) depression with cardiovascular collapse and respiratory failure. All of the drugs mentioned can have serious side effects. Diazepam (Valium) may be highly addictive. It is a controlled substance under federal law. Valium can be a tranquilizer (a drug that has a calming effect and is used to treat anxiety and emotional tension).

Dantrolene has a probability to cause liver damage. The incidence of hepatitis is related to the amount of drug that you have taken, but may occur even with a short period of small doses. Hepatitis has been most frequently observed between the third and twelfth months of therapy. The risk of liver injury appears to be greater in women, in patients over 35 years of age and in patients taking other medications in addition to dantrolene.

If you are taking certain muscle relaxants and experience a purple colored urine, you do not have a serious illness. For example, methocarbamol and chlorzoxazone may cause harmless color changes in your urine such as orange or reddish-purple with chlorzoxazone and purple, brown, or green with methocarbamol. Your urine will return to its normal color when you stop taking the medicine. Because each of these drugs can cause sedation, they should be used with caution with other drugs including alcohol that may also cause drowsiness. Drugs that inhibit the metabolism of Valium in your liver may increase the activity of the diazepam (Valium). These drugs include: cimetidine, oral contraceptives, disulfiram, fluoxetine, isoniazid, ketoconazole, metoprolol, propoxyphene, propranolol, and valproic acid. In females dantrolene may have an interaction with estrogens. The rate of liver damage in women over the age of 35 who were taking estrogens is higher than in other groups.

14. Antiinflammatory Medications

RSD/CRPS is an inflammatory disease. As a result many patients are prescribed nonsteroidal anti-inflammatory drugs. Cyclooxygenase, an enzyme involved in inflammation can be inhibited by antiinflammatory drugs like ibuprofen. Cyclooxygenase-2 has been implicated in the development of RSD/CRPS. Steroids are drugs used to reduce inflammatory pain such as arthritic joint pain. However, steroids may have significant side effects associated with their use. For example, steroids can cause weight gain, osteoporosis, avascular necrosis of your hips etc. Nonsteroidal anti-inflammatory drugs are commonly used to treat painful conditions. These may include a sprain strain injury, a headache, a toothache etc. M any individuals believe that these drugs are safe because many of them are sold over the counter. However, these drugs may have serious side effects in some individuals.

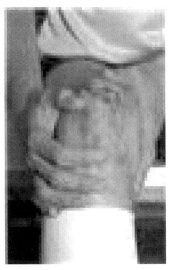

Figure 1. Nonsteroidal anti-inflammatory drugs are useful in a variety of bone, joint, tendon and muscle pain. These medications may also be useful in the treatment of pain caused be RSD/CRPS.

The first type of painkillers that are often used to treat the pain of RSD/CRPS are nonsteroidal anti-inflammatory drugs (NSAIDs), such as ibuprofen. People are often surprised that their use is recommended to treat severe pain, but they have proved to be very effective in relieving the symptoms of RSD/CRPS in many people. They can also help to reduce any associated swelling and may help relieve pain and redness.

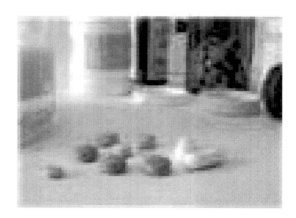

Figure 2.. There are many different types of NSAIDS. If one type does not provide you with pain relief, another type may provide you with pain relief.

Nonsteroidal anti-inflammatory drugs inhibit prostaglandins. Prostagland-ins are a related family of chemicals that are produced by the cells of your body and have several important functions. They promote inflammation, pain, and cause fevers. They are involved with the function of platelets that are necessary for the clotting of your blood, and protect the lining of your stomach from the damaging effects of acid. Prostaglandins are produced within your body's cells by the enzyme cyclooxygenase (COX). There are two of these enzymes, COX 1 and COX 2. However, only COX-1 produces prostaglandins that support platelets and protect the stomach. Nonsteroidal anti-inflammatory drugs (NSAIDs) block the COX enzymes and reduce prostaglandins throughout your body. As a consequence, ongoing inflammation, pain, and fever are reduced. Since the prostagland-ins that protect the stomach and support the platelets and blood clotting also are reduced, NSAIDs can cause ulcers in your the stomach and cause bleeding. NSAIDs differ in how strongly they inhibit COX-1 and, there-fore, in their tendency to cause ulcers and promote bleeding.

Another important difference between the two enzymes is their ability to cause ulcers and bleeding. The more an NSAID blocks COX-1, the greater is its tendency to cause ulcers and bleeding. One NSAID called Celebrex, blocks COX-2, but has little effect on COX-1. This drug is referred to as one of the selective COX-2 inhibitors and therefore causes less bleeding and fewer ulcers than other NSAIDs. Aspirin is the only NSAID that is able to inhibit the clotting of blood for a prolonged period (4 to 7 days). This prolonged effect of aspirin makes it an ideal drug for preventing the blood clots that cause heart attacks and strokes. COX-2 inhibitors do not cause your blood to not clot. This is one reason why COX-2 inhibitors are implicated in heart attacks. You should be aware that the FDA issued a public health advisory concerning use of non-steroidal anti-inflammatory drug products including those known as COX-2 selective agents. The COX-2 selective agents like Celebrex may be associated with an increased risk of serious cardiovascular events especially when they are used for long periods of time or in very high-risk settings. The drugs Vioxx and Bextra have been taken off the market. Preliminary results from a long-term clinical trial suggest that long-term use of a non-selective NSAID; naproxen may be associated with an increased cardiovascular risk compared to placebo. Celebrex and other anti-inflammatory coxib medications may counter the positive effects of aspirin in preventing blood clots.

The research, published in the Proceedings of the National Academy of Sciences (PNAS), indicates that people who are taking aspirin and coxibs together are in fact inhibiting the aspirin's effectiveness in preventing heart attacks and strokes. It is suggested that patients who are consuming coxibs and a low dose of aspirin simultaneously are exposed to a greater risk of cardiovascular events. In the past decade, a new group of anti-inflammatory drugs, coxibs, which include Celebrex was developed to treat arthritic pain as well as other pain such as RSD/CRPS. Arthritis patients who take Celebrex are instructed to take low-dose aspirin to counteract Celebrex's own potential clot-promoting effect.

Aspirin is the oldest and one of the most effective non steroidal anti-inflammatory drugs. It is also well known for its ability to prevent the blood clots that can potentially lead to heart attack and stroke. Therefore, doctors often advise patients who are more prone to heart-related illnesses to take a daily tablet of low dose aspirin (81 mg). Approximately, 50 million Americans take aspirin every day to reduce their risk of cardiovascular diseases.

The FDA (Federal Drug Administration) stated that patients who are at a high risk of gastrointestinal bleeding, have a history of intolerance to non-selective NSAIDs, or are not doing well on non-selective NSAIDs may be appropriate candidates for COX-2 selective agents. Non-selective NSAIDs are widely used in both over-the-counter and prescription settings. As prescription drugs, many are approved for short-term use in the treatment of pain and menstrual discomfort, and for longer-term use to treat the signs and symptoms of osteoarthritis and rheumatoid arthritis. NSAIDS are classified as non-opioid analgesic drugs and are aspirin like drugs. Although the pharmacologic and toxicologic properties of these compounds are similar and all possess analgesic activity, only certain drugs are indicated specifically for the relief of pain (eg. Feldene, Voltaren, Advil, Naprosyn, Celebrex etc,). NSAIDS stop the production of prostaglandin production. Since prostaglandins are formed and released in response to cell membrane injury, these substances have become associated with pain reactions that accompany tissue injury and inflammation. Prostaglandins sensitize pain receptors (mostly C fibers) by lowering the threshold to thermal, mechanical and chemical stimuli.

Thus, the increased pain sensations induced by prostaglandins is a localized event that allows the mediators of pain such as bradykinin, histamine and substance P, to exert a greater effect on pain receptors. The receptors are stimulated to a greater extent causing more pain. All of the NSAIDS analgesics prevent the biosynthesis and release of prostaglandins by inhibition of prostaglandin cyclooxygenase, a cell membrane enzyme that is present in almost all cells. Therefore, the NSAIDS reduce the formation of prostaglandins and decrease the pain sensitivity caused by these substances. NSAIDS have analgesic, fever reducing, and anti-inflammatory effects.

Not all of the drugs are equally active, nor are all clinically useful, with respect to these effects. Dolobid (diflunisal) for example, is used exclusively as an analgesic but does not decrease a fever. With the exception of acetaminophen, aspirin, and ibuprofen, none of the other compounds are used to reduce fever. NSAIDS are used in the treatment of various arthritic conditions such as rheumatoid arthritis, ankylosing spondylitis, osteoarthritis and acute gouty arthritis. As the particular inflammatory condition being treated is alleviated, the pain associated with the disease is also decreased. Pain associated with inflammatory diseases is effectively reduced by all of these NSAID drugs. Aspirin is the oldest NSAID.

Toradol (ketolorac) has minimal antiinflammatory effects but has significant pain relieving effects. This observation suggests that antiinflammatory effects are not related to pain relieving effects. NSAIDS have a ceiling affect. This means that when you take a certain dose of an NSAID, more of the NSAID will not give you more pain relief. This affect is opposite to that of opioid analgesics. They have no ceiling effects. This means that more of an opioid will increase your pain relief. Research studies have concluded that IV parecoxib is an effective antiinflammatory drug combined with clonidine/lidocaine loco-regional block in RSD/CRPS type 1. However, the FDA will not permit this drug to be marketed.

In some cases of RSD/CRPS anti-inflammatory agents have no effects on RSD/CRPS pain. These results indicate a non-inflammatory pathogenesis in RSD/CRPS presumably central in origin. The Bayer Company in Germany discovered aspirin in the late 1800's. Aspirin is the prototype to which other NSAIDS are compared. The side effects of the NSAIDS should be briefly discussed. Serious side effects are rare. The liver and kidneys can be affected by high doses of NSAIDS prescribed over a long duration. Patients with forms of arthritis will require NSAIDS long term for the anti-inflammatory properties of the NSAIDS.

Gastrointestinal toxicity can occur with all NSAIDS that can lead to bleeding from the stomach and may lead to hospitalization and surgery as well as blood transfusions. Localized irritation of the stomach lining constitutes the most common adverse reaction associated NSAIDS. Although epigastric distress is common at the lower doses, gastric and/or intestinal ulceration and bleeding will occur in only a small percentage of patients. At higher doses of aspirin, erosive gastritis and gastrointestinal hemorrhage is observed more often. These effects are the result of the inhibition of cyclooxygenase 1 (COX-1). You need cyclooxygenase 1 to form protective prostaglandins that reduce acid secretion by your stomach and promote the secretion of protective intestinal mucus. Aspirin and other compounds with high anti-inflammatory activity, such as indomethacin, tend to elicit the highest incidence of gastrointestinal reactions. Other NSAIDS like naproxen are considered to produce fewer and less intense gastrointestinal reactions than aspirin.

Acetaminophen is essentially devoid of these effects. Acetaminophen has some anti-inflammatory affects. Newer NSAIDS that are specific for cyclo oxygenase 2 enzymes are safer than the rest of the NSAIDS that inhibit both cyclooxygenase 1 and 2. Celebrex is safer on your stomach. With respect to the heart and lungs all of the NSAIDS can cause swelling in your extremities as well as increase your blood pressure.

It should be noted that all NSAIDS including ibuprofen and naproxen could be linked to an increased risk of a heart attack. Because of this research, it is advisable to use the lowest effective dose of NSAID for the shortest time necessary, NSAIDS can cause clotting problems and make you prone to bleeding or bruising. This is due to the inhibition of thromboxane A, formation in thrombocytes (cells in the bloodstream associated with clotting). However, Celebrex does not cause this problem. In other words, Celebrex is the only NSAID that does not adversely affect the blood thinning effects of aspirin.

With respect to your kidneys, sodium and water retention with extremity swelling are seen with NSAID use. The higher the dose, the more prone you are for these side effects. Ask your doctor about the lowest effective dose that can be prescribed for you. If you are over sixty years of age you should be prescribed lower doses, as you may be more sensitive to NSAIDS than younger patients. NSAIDS are excellent analgesic medications for pain in extremities, as well as for dental pain and headaches. They are furthermore, non addicting. NSAIDS should be used with caution in elderly patients. If you are significantly sick (such as an intensive care patient, an NSAID can adversely affect your kidneys. In some instances NSAIDS can cause kidney failure.

Nonsteroidal anti-inflammatory drugs (NSAIDs) are commonly used in the elderly for the treatment of fever, pain, pain associated with inflammation in rheumatoid arthritis and osteoarthritis, neuromuscular disorders, headache, and musculoskeletal conditions. Each year in the United States, people spend 5 to 10 billion dollars to purchase prescription and over-the-counter NSAIDs. Gastrointestinal side effects such as ulcers and bleeding are the most prevalent and life-threatening problems associated with NSAIDs in elderly individuals. Specifically in the elderly, NSAIDs have become a leading cause of hospitalization in this age group and may increase the risk of death from ulceration more than four fold. NSAIDs and the new class of cyclo-oxygenase-2 selective NSAIDs continue as drugs of choice for analgesia and anti-inflammatory effects. Physiological changes of aging worsen the side-effect profile of NSAIDs in the elderly. These side effects, when added to the increased potential for drug interactions, lead to a much greater risk for adverse outcomes when NSAIDs are used in the elderly patient.

NSAIDS should be used with caution in pregnant patients as well. These drugs are not recommended during pregnancy, especially in the third trimester. While NSAIDs as a class are not direct congenital malformation drugs. They may however, cause premature closure of the fetal ductus arteriosus and also cause a reduction in maternal amniotic fluid. As a result, pregnant patients taking NSAIDS may require ultrasound monitoring by the treating obstetrician. In addition NSAIDS may cause premature birth. Aspirin should not be used during pregnancy. Fetal bleeding could occur as a result of the inhibitory effects on the fetal platelets. Acetaminophen which does have slight anti-inflammatory properties is safe and well-tolerated during pregnancy.

15. Opioid Medications

Narcotic drugs may be ineffective for the management of RSD/CRPS pain. RSD/CRPS pain is called neuropathic pain meaning nerve fiber pain. Narcotic drugs on the other hand, are prescribed for postoperative pain, cancer pain and for some chronic pain syndromes. Narcotic drugs can relieve moderate to severe pain. The term narcotic refers to agents that benumb or deaden nerves, causing loss of feeling or paralysis. Psychodelic drugs like LSD, contrary to popular belief are not narcotics. Many law enforcement officials in the United States inaccurately use the word "narcotic" to refer to any illegal drug or any unlawfully possessed drug. Some physicians prescribe narcotics for RSD/CRPS pain. It has been stated that neuropathic pain is less sensitive to opioids, meaning higher doses are required compared to known non-neuropathic pain. Thus, observation that higher doses of opioids are needed in neuropathic pain to provide pain relief has been confirmed by many studies. demonstrated that higher doses of narcotics produce a better effect on pain relief in neuropathic pain.

Most medical professionals prefer the term opioid which refers to natural, semi-synthetic and synthetic substances that behave pharmacologically like morphine. The Opioids are a class of controlled pain-management drugs that contain natural or synthetic chemicals based on morphine, the active component of opium. These narcotics effectively mimic the pain-relieving chemicals that the body produces naturally. Opioids are the most often prescribed pain-relievers because they are so effective. Morphine is the standard to which other opioid drugs are compared. Morphine is frequently prescribed to alleviate severe pain after surgery. Codeine can be helpful in soothing somewhat milder pain, as are oxycodone (OxyContin, an oral, controlled-release form of the drug), propoxyphene (Darvon), hydrocodone (Vicodin), hydromorphone (Dilaudid) and meperidine (Demerol), which is used less often because of its side effects. Diphenoxylate or Lomotil can also relieve severe diarrhea, and codeine can ease severe coughs.

The primary medical use of opioids is to relieve pain. Other medical uses include control of coughs and diarrhea, and the treatment of addiction to other opioids. Opioids can produce euphoria, making them prone to abuse. Opioids should only be used for moderate to severe pain that has not responded to non-narcotic drugs like aspirin or ibuprofen.

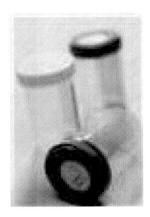

Figure 1. There are many types of narcotic medications. You may need to try more than one narcotic medication before you obtain pain relief.

Narcotics can be used alone like oxycodone or used in combination with aspirin, ibuprofen or acetaminophen (Tylenol). Some narcotics like oxycodone or morphine are available as an extended release tablet that must be swallowed whole. Tablets, which are not extended release, may be split. In 1914, the Federal Government passed a law that prohibited prescribing opioid drugs for recreational use. The Federal Controlled Substances Act of 1970 formulated schedules for drugs. You need to be aware of three of five schedules; I, has no current accepted medical use like heroin or marijuana, II; high abuse and dependence potential like morphine, codeine or oxycodone, and III; includes drugs with a lesser dependence and abuse liability. Hydrocodone (Vicodin) is a schedule III drug. Valium, a relaxant is a schedule IV drug and some cough medicines are schedule V drugs. Oxycodone (Oxycotin) is a schedule II drug which means that it is potentially more habit forming than hydrocodone.

There is a difference between the descriptions of narcotic drugs and opioids. Opioids are drugs like morphine, hydrocodone etc. Narcotics are extremely addictive drugs and include heroin and other drugs that can cause sedation. Opioids act by attaching to a group of proteins called opioid receptors, found in the brain, spinal cord and gastrointestinal tract.

When these drugs link to certain opioid receptors in the brain and spinal cord they can block the transmission of pain messages to the brain.

For the purposes of discussion in outlining the pharmacologic activity of these compounds, the opioids will be classified as (1) agonists, (2) antagonists, and (3) mixed agonist-antagonists. All drugs bind to receptors that exist on the outer membrane of your cells. Narcotics bind to narcotic receptors on cells in the brain and spinal cord. Opioid receptors may also be recruited on tissue cells outside of your central nervous system such as your knee following an injury. An injection of morphine into your knee may alleviate your pain. When opioids turn on a receptor, that receptor decreases pain signals usually in your spinal cord that prevents pain signals from going to your brain. As a result, your pain perception is decreased. Experimental studies involving binding of opioids to specific receptors in the brain and spinal cord have substantiated the hypothesis that these receptors exist which mediates the actions of the opioid drugs to stop pain signals to your brain.

There are two basic classes of opioid receptors called mu and kappa receptors. Other classes exist (e.g. delta) but are not important for the discussion of your pain in this chapter. These receptors also appear to be the site of action of the endogenous (pain drugs produced by your body) opioid-like substances and have been divided into three major categories, designated mu, and kappa. It has also been proposed that at least two subtypes of each category of opioid receptors exist. Experimental evidence suggests that activation of mu receptors (found principally at sites in the brain) is associated with analgesia, respiratory depression, euphoria, and physical dependence. The kappa receptors (located within the spinal cord) are believed to mediate spinal analgesia, constriction of the pupil size and sedation.

The other receptors may influence affective behavior, and although some physicians believe that activation of these receptors plays a role in opioid-induced analgesia, this remains controversial. Since a number of different compounds, (e.g., certain antihistamines, some steroids, and anti psychotics have phencyclidine) none of which are opioid in structure but can affect binding affinity for these sites. Agonistic (stimulating) opioids act as analgesics by binding to and activating both mu and kappa receptors in the brain and spinal cord. The opioid antagonists bind to all categories of opioid receptor sites throughout the body, but fail to activate them. These compounds are not used for pain control; rather, the utility of these drugs lies in their ability to reverse an overdose of opioids including narcotics.

The compounds that comprise the mixed agonist-antagonist group are more recent additions to the clinically important opioids. These drugs are semi-synthetic derivatives of morphine, the chemical structures of which have agonistic activity at some kappa receptors but antagonistic activity at mu receptors, e.g., pentazocine, butorphanol, and nalbuphine, or partial agonistic activity at mu receptors and antagonistic activity at kappa receptors, eg. buprenorphine. All are effective analgesics since they stimulate either mu or kappa receptors. The use of pain medication in long term pain narcotic patients should be limited to the non-addicting type of pain medications (such as Stadol or Ultram) or to the less addicting pain medications such as Nubane and Talacen.

Chemically, the opioid agonists include a number of classes of drugs, all of which have pharmacologic effects similar to those of morphine. Morphine is the oldest known drug of this class. It remains as the prototype for the opioid group and is the standard to which all other opioid analgesic drugs are compared. Opioid drugs decrease pain but also affect all organ systems. Your pituitary gland in your brain can be adversely affected by chronic narcotic use. For example in males opioids can decrease testosterone that can cause depression and erectile dysfunction. Drowsiness and blurred vision can occur. Changes in mood can occur. An inability to concentrate can occur.

Euphoria can be experienced in 20% of individuals taking opioid drugs. Euphoria can be the cause of addiction. Opioids can stop your respiratory drive that can cause you to stop breathing. Narcotics affect your stomach by slowing down the passage of food in combination with your brain to cause nausea and vomiting. Opioids can cause a significant decrease in your blood pressure that may cause you to fall. Opioids decrease movement of the bowel resulting in constipation. Morphine can make gall bladder disease worse by contracting a valve where the gall bladder meets the intestine called the sphincter of Oddi. Opioid drugs can result in a release of histamine from certain cell in the body that can cause itching and a rash. As you can see opioid drugs can have side effects.

Tolerance, addiction and physical dependence can occur with opioid drugs. Tolerance occurs when it takes more drug to cause the same decrease in your pain. This is not addiction. Patients may find that they develop tolerance to opioid pain medications and may need to have their doses increased in order to be effective. Tolerance has not been shown to lead to drug addiction. Physical dependence is a condition that occurs when continued use of the drug is needed to prevent a withdrawal reaction. Steady use of opioids can result in tolerance to the drugs so that higher doses must be taken to achieve the same effects. Long-term use also can lead to physical dependence—the body adapts to the presence of the drug and withdrawal symptoms occur if use is reduced abruptly.

Addiction is an intense craving for an opioid and is often associated with recreational use. Signs and symptoms of addiction include yawning, sweating, restlessness, irritability, anxiety, nasal discharge, tearing, dilated pupils, gooseflesh, tremors, loss of appetite, body aches, nausea and vomiting, fever and chills and an increase in heart rate and blood pressure. These symptoms last 7-10 days. Minor symptoms can begin in 8-12 hours after the last dose of the opioid. The more severe symptoms like nausea and vomiting begin 48-72 hours after the last dose of the drug.

With respect to agonist drugs, morphine is the prototype. It can be administered by mouth, rectum or by injection into muscle or vein. Is is prepared in a capsule, tablet or a liquid. It is available by a rectal supository as well. This route of administration is used for those patients who cannot swallow or are having severe vomiting. Hydromorphone and oxymorphone also come in the form of rectal suppositories. The duration of action of opioids varies from drug to drug. Sustained release morphine and oxycodone give a longer duration of action. Immediate release drugs (eg. OXIR) give a faster onset but have a shorter duration of action. Fentanyl, which is 75 times more potent than morphine is available in a patch and sucker, forms. The fentanyl patch is used for severe constant pain. The pain relief is continuous. The sucker, which only comes in a raspberry flavor, is used for severe cancer pain in instances where the severe pain fluctuates. Fentora is another oral form of fentanyl.

With respect to the fentanyl pain patch, the amount of drug released is controlled by small holes in a membrane in the patch. A larger hole permits the release of fentanyl into your body. The patches are available in different doses. The fentanyl is released for 48-72 hours. Patients with a fever can be at a risk for an overdose as the amount of fentanyl administered to your body can increase by 25% for every 30C increase in body temperature. The advantage of the patch is that patients do not have to take frequent pills during the night. The patch should be applied to a hairless surface.

The Food & Drug Administration recently granted marketing approval to oxymorphone immediate-release and oxymorphone extended-release tablets (Opana/Opana ER, Endo Pharmaceuticals). Opana is approved for relief of moderate to severe acute pain where the use of an opioid is appropriate. Opana ER is approved for relief of moderate to severe pain in patients requiring round-the-clock opioid treatment for an extended period. This approval marks the first time oxymorphone will be available in an oral and extended-release formulation. Opana ER is now available in most retail pharmacies.

"Opana ER represents a new member in a group of long-acting opioids now considered the standard of care for the treatment of chronic, non-cancer pain," said Russell Portenoy, M.D., chairman, Department of Pain Medicine and Palliative Care at Beth Israel Medical Center in New York City. "The immediate-release formulations are often used to treat break-through pain in combination with a long-acting opioid".

"This approval makes available an opioid not used previously for the management of chronic pain," said Portenoy. Individuals respond differently to each of the opioid analgesics, and we may need to rotate opioids in order to identify the compound that produces the most favorable ratio of analgesia to adverse effect, he said. "We can easily incorporate oral oxymorphone into this process of opioid rotation." The adverse-effect profiles of Opana and Opana ER are comparable to those of other opioids, he said. Darvon (propoxyphene) and codeine are weaker opioids that are used to treat mild pain. Darvon has been taken off the market because of its adverse affects on some patients hearts. They may be combined with acetaminophen to make each more potent. You need to be aware that smoking tobacco can decrease the potency of Darvon and hydrocodone.

Tramadol (Ultram) is an interesting drug and may be used for moderate to moderately severe pain. It has a low abuse potential. It is not a scheduled drug. It activates mu and kappa receptors. The side effects are minimal when compared to opioid drugs. Tramadol does not produce withdrawal symptoms like opioids. The advantage of tramadol over other drugs is that tramadol inhibits noreoinepherine and serotonin release from your brain and spinal cord. The two substances in the brain and spinal cord also decrease pain. The opioid drugs do not have this effect. Tramadol can cause nausea dizziness and headaches. Tramadol does not lower the heart rate or blood pressure. Tramadol provides pain relief similar to codeine and propoxyphene. Ryzolt (tramadol hydrochloride extended-release tablets) is a centrally acting analgesic composed of a dual-matrix delivery system with both immediate-release and extended-release characteristics.

Naloxone and naltrexone are drugs that reverse the respiratory effects of opioids. Naltrexone can be given orally. The only time that these drugs are given is to treat opioid intoxication. Butorphanol (Stadol) and pentazocine (Talwin) are called mixed agonist-antagonists drugs. These drugs show receptor selectivity and these two drugs stimulate kappa receptors. These drugs have less opioid abuse tendencies than the agonist drugs. Opioids on the other hand work on both mu and kappa receptors. Strong opioids exist which are usually reserved for cancer patients or other patients with severe pain.

Hydromorphone (Dilaudid) and levorphanol (Levo-Droman) are eight and five times more potent than morphine. Meperidine (Demerol) is an opioid that is weaker than morphine. It is used infrequently in pain management as it can cause tremors or seizures if used on a chronic basis. Methadone is a synthetic drug similar to morphine. The advantage of methadone for your pain management is that it does not cause euphoria. Methadone however, can cause a conduction problem in your heart. Consequently, patients have died from heart problems after being pre-scribed methadone. Hydrocodone and oxycodone are two opioids used for moderate to moderately severe pain. These drugs are usually combined with aspirin and acetaminophen which can potentiate the analgesic efficacy of these drugs.

In some individuals some narcotic drugs do not provide pain relief. This happens in 20-30% of paients. This is because some narcotics like hydrocodone, codeine, oxycodone and tramadol need to be converted by an enzyme in your body called CYP 34A. The drugs themselves only decrease pain after each is converted to another chemical in your body. The drug that you are prescribed is converted to a pain relieving drug in your body. For example, hydrocodone is converted to morphine. The morphine provides you pain relief, not the hydrocodone itself.

If you have a genetic abnormality, the CYP 450 enzyme does not convert hydrocodone to morphine. Therefore, you feel no pain relief. Antidepressant drugs, benzodiazepine drugs like Valium can inhibit the cyrochrome p 450 enzyme which in turn inhibits the CYP 34A enzyme. Drugs like fentanyl, morphone dilaudid and oxymorphone do not need this enzyme activity to provide pain relief. Many patients are terminated from pain practices because their narcotics like hydrocodone provide no pain relief. Some doctors unfortunately believe that the patients are drug seeking and the doctors terminate patients from their practice.

Another fact that you need to know is that opioid drugs can actually cause you to experience increased pain in some instances. This observation is called opioid induced pain. Many physicians are unaware of this fact. In this situation, a reduction in your dose of your medicine or stopping it can actually decrease your pain. This phenomenon can also be seen in patents who have spinal morphine drug delivery systems. Another fact that you need to be aware of is that smoking cigarettes can affect the absorption of some narcotics from your stomach to your blood stream. Drugs have to get to your brain to become effective for pain relief.

As one can see, there are many opioids that can be used for the management of your acute chronic pain. The proper choice of your medication is dependent upon the magnitude of your pathology, the side effects of the drug prescribed, the effectiveness of the drug and your overall health. In general, opioids are not always useful for the management of RSD/CRPS pain because RSD/CRPS is primarily nerve pain. However, when bone, muscles and ligaments are involved in an injury, narcotic drugs may be indicated.

16. Addiction

Drugs are chemicals that have a profound impact on the neurochemical balance in your brain. This action affects how you feel and act. People who are suffering emotionally use drugs to escape from their problems. This can lead to drug abuse and addiction. Some physicians are afraid to prescribe scheduled drugs because of the possibility of causing addiction. Addiction is a chronic relapsing brain disease. Brain imaging shows that addiction severely alters your brain areas critical to decision-making, learning and memory, and behavior control, which may help to explain the compulsive and destructive behaviors of addiction. An addiction is a recurring problem by an individual to engage in some specific activity, despite harmful consequences to the individual's health, mental state or social life. An addiction can occur with drugs, gambling, overeating etc. Drugs can make you euphoric. As a result, you may request more and more drugs to maintain this euphoria.

Drug abuse or substance abuse, involves the repeated and excessive use of prescription or street drugs. In one way or another, almost all drugs over stimulate the pleasure center of the brain, flooding it with the neurotransmitter dopamine which produces euphoria. That heightened sense of pleasure can be so compelling that the brain wants that feeling back, again and again. Addiction is frequently found in people with a wide variety of mental illnesses, including anxiety disorders, unipolar and bipolar depression, schizophrenia, and borderline and other personality disorders. Methadone can be used for the treatment of pain in addicted patients. Methadone is also an opiate that prevents users from getting high on heroin by competing with the much more potent opiates for the body's opiate receptors. Buprenophrine is another drug that is effective for the treatment of addiction and is also an analgesic.

Addiction and drug dependence occur when drugs become so important that you are willing to sacrifice your work, home and even your family. Once your brain and body get used to the substances you are taking, you begin to require increasingly larger and more frequent doses, in order to achieve the same effect. Narcotics such as Heroin may over-stimulate the pleasure centers of the brain producing euphoric effects that cause compulsive drug-seeking behaviors. The severities of withdrawal symptoms associated with narcotics include chills, shakes, muscle pain, nausea, vomiting, and headaches and cravings.

A clinician must be able to distinguish between legitimate patients with chronic pain and individuals engaged in non-therapeutic drug seeking behavior. Physicians have for years recognized the value of opioid analgesics in relieving chronic pain. Unfortunately, drug seekers may also request opioid analgesics. They do this by feigning illnesses, and seek controlled substances from multiple doctors and by forge prescriptions. Drug seekers may be difficult to distinguish from true chronic pain sufferers. In general, drug seekers prefer illicit drugs such as heroin and cocaine to prescription drugs.

Prescription drugs however, have advantages over illicit drugs. Third-party insurers or welfare-entitlement programs may pay for prescribed drugs. Prescription pharmaceuticals are obtained in the safety of the physician's office. Drug abuse and addiction have a devastating impact on society. Heroin use alone is responsible for the epidemic number of new cases of HIV/AIDS and hepatitis. Drug abuse is responsible for decreased job productivity and attendance, increased healthcare costs, and an escalation of domestic violence and violent crimes.

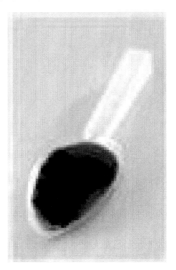

Figure 1. Drug addiction is a serious public health problem in the United States.

An estimated 20 percent of people in the United States have used prescription drugs for nonmedical reasons. Central nervous stimulants, depressants and opioids are prescription drugs that are frequently abused. Central nervous system depressants are used to treat anxiety, panic attacks, and sleep disorders. Examples are Nembutal (pentobarbital sodium), Valium (diazepam), and Xanax (alprazolam). Long-term use can lead to physical dependence and addiction. Central nervous system stimulants are used to treat narcolepsy and the attention-deficit/hyperactivity disorder. Examples include Ritalin (methylphenidate) and Dexedrine (dextroamphetamine). Opioids, also known as narcotic analgesics are used to treat pain. Opioids are the most commonly abused prescription drugs. Examples include morphine, codeine, OxyContin (oxycodone), Vicodin (hydrocodone) and Demerol (meperidine).

One may obtain drugs by the following means: prescription forgery, by telephone (faking to be a physician's office), multiple doctors, and indiscriminate prescribing by physicians. Pain clinicians who prescribe chronic opioids are aware that there is an illicit market for opioid analgesics. For example Oxycontin can be sold for $1.00 per milligram. One 80 mg pill can be sold on the street for $80.00. Telephone scams occur when the drug seeker claims to be a patient of one of the other physicians in the on-call group, and asks for a prescription for an analgesic to last until they can see their regular physician. Sometimes, the drug seeker uses a telephone to impersonate a practicing physician.

Prescription forgery is a common activity among drug seekers. Drug seekers can modify a legitimate prescription to increase the dosage or quantity of an opioid. The easiest method is to increase the number of tablets on the prescription. Multiple episodes of noncompliance raise an alert of drug seeking behavior as well as multiple episodes of prescription loss. The patient with chemical dependency loses control over drug taking. The patient cannot take medications as prescribed. The patient repeatedly reports lost or stolen medications.

The physician will notice that the drug seeker frequently requests early renewals of prescriptions. A pain physician must however, be aware that aggressive complaining about the need for more drugs may indicate inadequate pain management as opposed to drug seeking behavior. A patient should not be allowed to suffer. It should be understood that substance abusers can suffer from chronic pain which should be treated in a humane manner. Unapproved use of opioids to treat another symptom such as sleep deprivation should not be tolerated. However, the pain management physician must objectively identify a patient's pain complaint with the appropriate medical test before prescribing an opioid. Opioid analgesics are powerful tools in the armamentarium of the pain clinician. Criminal and chemically dependent drug seekers may attempt to obtain such drugs from the physician. A pain medicine physician must therefore, use safe prescribing strategies. A physician has no legal obligation to prescribe opioid analgesics on demand. A reasonable precaution to be taken by the pain medicine physician with an unfamiliar patient is to establish a policy of not prescribing opioid analgesics pending a complete assessment including corroboration of the patient's history. Some patients or patient families are afraid of addiction. However, a significant number of individuals do not understand the difference between addiction and tolerance.

The American Academy of Pain Medicine, the American Pain Society, and the American Society of Addiction Medicine recognize the following definitions and recommend their use.

I.Addiction

Addiction is a primary, chronic, neurobiologic disease, with genetic, psychosocial, and environmental factors influencing its development and manifestations. It is characterized by behaviors that include one or more of the following: impaired control over drug use, compulsive use, continued use despite harm, and craving. An entity termed pseudo-addiction exists which is not true addiction. Pseudo-addiction occurs when pain is under treated. Pseudoaddiction resolves when the pain resolves. Addictive behavior on the other hand, persists in spite of increasing the patient's pain medication.

II. Physical Dependence

Physical dependence is a state of adaptation that is manifested by a drug class specific withdrawal syndrome that can be produced by abrupt cessation, rapid dose reduction, decreasing blood level of the drug, and/or administration of an antagonist.

III. Tolerance

Tolerance is a state of adaptation in which exposure to a drug induces changes that result in a   diminution of one or more of the drug's effects over time. Most specialists in pain medicine and addiction medicine agree that patients treated with prolonged opioid therapy usually do develop physical dependence and sometimes develop tolerance, but do not usually develop addictive disorders. Addiction is a primary chronic disease and exposure to opioid medications is only one of the etiologic factors in its development. Therefore, good clinical judgment must be used in determining whether the pattern of behaviors signals the presence of addiction or reflects a different issue.

17. Morphine Spinal Pumps

Narcotic drugs like morphine, baclofen, a muscle relaxant and a snail toxin called Prialt can be administered into your spinal fluid for RSD/CRPS pain control. A long term spinal fluid morphine therapy is a useful treatment option for patients with intractable severe RSD/CRPS who have failed other therapies and remain markedly disabled. Patients with a chronic regional pain syndrome (CRPS) can find some relief with a series of somatic and sympatholytic blockades, which allow an aggressive physiotherapy once the pain is under control. Drugs are administered via a pump system from a pump placed in your stomach area with a tube that goes to your spinal fluid. The spinal infusion pump, commonly known as a "morphine pump", is a specialized device, which delivers concentrated amounts of medication into the spinal fluid space via a small catheter (Figure 1.). The intrathecal space is the sac that contains the spinal fluid. The spinal infusion pump is also identified as an intrathecal infusion pump. Spinal infusion pump implants are offered to patients with chronic and severe pain, who have not adequately responded to other, more conservative, treatments. Usually these patients cannot be easily controlled on oral pain medications. As a result, to control their pain, these patients may benefit from a continuous spinal infusion of a pain medication, like morphine. Patients have to meet certain screening criteria before a spinal infusion pump is implanted.

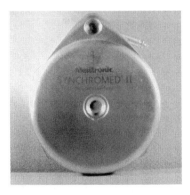

Figure 1. Spinal pump. The center of the pump has a hole where a drug can be placed to give you continual pain relief. The pump is battery

driven and the dose of drug administered is controlled by a hand held programmer.

The spinal infusion pump delivers concentrated amounts of medication into the spinal fluid, thus continuously bathing the pain receptors on the spinal cord with pain medication. This allows the patient to eliminate or substantially decrease the need for oral medications for pain control. The pump system delivers medication around the clock, thus eliminating or minimizing breakthrough pain and other symptoms. The implantation of a spinal infusion pump is a surgical procedure. The patient procedure involves inserting an introducer needle through skin and deeper tissues. So, there is some pain involved. However, the skin and deeper tissues are numbed with a local anesthetic using a very thin needle before inserting the larger introducer needle. Almost all of the patients have anesthesia or also receive deep intravenous sedation that makes the procedure easy to tolerate. The spinal infusion catheter is inserted in the midline at the lower back. The infusion pump is then placed on the side of the abdomen in a pocket under the skin.

The pump is usually activated while you are still on the operating table. There will typically be some swelling over the pump site and tenderness or pain from the incisions. However, in many patients, this surgical pain and tenderness is controlled by the morphine infusion and may not require additional pain medications. The medication contained within the pump will last about 1 to 3 months depending upon the concentration and amount infused. It is then refilled via a tiny needle inserted into the pump chamber. This is done in the office or at your home and it takes only a few minutes.

The batteries in the pump may last 3 to 5 years depending upon the usage. The batteries cannot be replaced or recharged. The pump must be replaced at that time. It is sometimes difficult to predict if a spinal infusion pump will indeed help you or not. For that reason a trial of different doses of morphine injection into the spine is carried out to determine if a permanent pump would be effective to relieve your pain or not. To find out whether a morphine pump is going to be effective, a trial with a temporary catheter connected to an externalized pump is often performed.

The Synchromed system is very expensive and you therefore want tp know if the spinal drug system will provide pain relief. The trial is performed as an in-patient. A narrow gauge temporary catheter is inserted into the intrathecal space in the operating theatre using local anesthetic and intravenous sedation. This catheter is then tunneled around to the front of the abdomen and fixed in place with a nurse-proof and patient-proof dressing. The catheter is then attached to an ambulatory battery operated infusion pump which contains the preservative free intrathecal (IT) morphine. During the first 24 hours the morphine-containing oral drugs are slowly stopped, while the intrathecal morphine infusion is gradually increased to the point where the only morphine received is via the intrathecal route.

All other pain killers which do not contain morphine may be continued as normal e.g. NSAIDs, amitriptyline, gabapentin etc. Mobilization is encouraged the day after the procedure, and is combined with IT morphine dose adjustments to achieve reasonable relief while fully ambulant. A successful trial is one where there is obvious improvement in pain relief during a full range of normal activities e.g. walking, sitting, dressing, bending etc. At the end of the trial, the temporary catheter is removed, after noting the 24 hour dose of IT morphine. This helps the implanting surgeon start at the correct dose immediately post procedure.

Other types of spinal trials have been described. A single shot injection of spinal morphine may be administered. the effect of the morphine lasts only 24 hours and does not allow an adequate trial of full mobilization. Spinal headaches can also occur. Epidural infusions may be tried. Achievement with an epidural infusion does not guarantee success with an IT infusion and vice versa. You should be aware that MRIs, if necessary, can be performed with a spinal infusion catheter and infusion pump in place. Special protocols for pump patients can be given to the MRI technicians and radiologists.

Prialt,(ziconotide) a snail toxin may help control pain from CRPS. This is a new drug used in the spinal drug delivery systems. Of the patients who experienced substantial improvement in pain, edema, skin abnormalities, and/or mobility with ziconotide therapy, some patients have discontinued ziconotide and are pain free. Other patients experienced marked reversal of both edema and advanced skin trophic changes. Adverse events included urinary retention, depression, anxiety, and hallucinations. Adverse events generally resolved spontaneously, with treatment, or with ziconotide discontinuation/dose reduction. Ziconotide holds promise as an effective treatment for RSD/CRPS.

In conclusion, spinal fluid drug delivery can provide relief in some situations where other modalities have failed.

18. Topical Medications

Pain relievers that can be applied directly to your skin are available for the control of a variety of your pain syndromes. These topical pain relievers are a noninvasive and convenient method for delivering pain-relieving medication to you. This is especially important and beneficial if you are not able to take medications by mouth. Topical pain relievers include complementary and alternative medications as well as conventional medications. Topical forms of analgesics, or pain relievers, have been used throughout human history. The use of ointments for medicinal purposes is mentioned in the Bible on many occasions. The purpose of a topical analgesic is to transmit a medication through your skin for the effect of pain relief. The amount of drug that actually gets through your skin is determined by the amount of pressure applied as you rub it over your skin, the area of your skin covered by the drug, the way in which the drug is dissolved, and the use of dressings over your skin. Analgesics are available in ointments, creams, and gels. They also may be placed in patches that may be applied to your skin.

Ointments are semisolid preparations that melt at body temperature and spread easily. Ointments are not routinely used in the practice of pain medicine unless the ointment is specially compounded by a pharmacy. Ointments are defined in three categories based on your skin penetration. One type of ointment does not penetrate beyond the external layer of your skin called the epidermis. Ointments of this class can be used for the treatment of sunburn. A second type of ointment penetrates to the internal layer of your skin called the dermis. The third type of ointment actually goes through your skin to the nerves and ligaments and in some instances into your bloodstream.

Substances applied on your skin can evaporate. You do not want your analgesic drug evaporating from your skin. Your pharmacist will add substances such as glycerin to the ointment to keep this evaporation from happening. Ointments can be prepared by your pharmacist or purchased over the counter or by prescription. Some ointment preparations will contain absorption enhancers. Absorption enhancers make it easier for the drug to be absorbed through your skin. Azone and DMSO can both enhance the absorption of ointments through your skin. Ointments should be packaged in tubes.

Creams are opaque, thick, liquid substances that consist of medications dissolved in a cream base that usually vanishes through the skin. They are less of a liquid consistency than ointments. The term cream is used to describe a soft type of preparation that is less affected by your body temperature than ointments. Gels are a delivery system that usually contain penetration enhancers and are usually used for administering anti-inflammatory medications. The anti-inflammatory medication must be absorbed through your skin to provide you with pain relief. Gels are useful treatment methods if you have arthritic and/or muscle pain. Gels usually are thicker than creams or ointments and are usually clear, unlike creams and ointments. The concentration of medication in gels is usually no greater than 2 percent. For example, lidocaine, which is a numbing medicine for the control of pain, is dispensed as a 2 percent gel. However, the cream is available in a 5 percent concentration. This is because medications are usually absorbed through the skin better if used in gel form. Gels usually have clarity and sparkle. They maintain their thickness even with an elevated body temperature. Some gels have been developed to be given nasally. Some drugs are absorbed better through the nose than through the skin. Gels are usually dispensed in tubes or squeeze bottles.

Another delivery system for analgesics is a transdermal patch, which contains medication that is transmitted directly through your skin. A patch containing a medication is placed on your skin and remains there for a specified time so that the drug within the patch can be delivered through your skin to your bloodstream. Local anesthetics such as lidocaine, capsaicin cream, and fentanyl (discussed in the narcotic drugs chapter), a potent opioid medication, are some of the medicines that can be delivered through your skin using a transdermal drug delivery system. These patches should be applied only to areas on your skin that have no blisters or open areas such as a cut. The patches are made of adhesive materials. You should not use the patch if you are allergic to some adhesives. With respect to the patches, the amount of drug that is absorbed from the patch is directly related to the length of the application of the patch, as well as the area of your skin to which it is applied.

The advantage of the patch is that it gives you a continuous flow of analgesic medications. When you take a pill, after it leaves your stomach or intestine and enters into your bloodstream, you receive a high concentration of the drug initially. As the drug is distributed to other tissues in your body, your blood level concentration of the drug decreases. Once your body breaks down the drug, you will no longer have an analgesic affect of that particular drug. However, when using a patch, you will have a continuous release of the drug from the patch into your bloodstream. You will have constant pain relief without the peaks and valleys of the drug concentration in your bloodstream associated with oral medications.

Natural compounds such as herbs or leaves and roots also can be used to treat your pain topically. Aloe vera can be used to decrease your pain if you have sunburn. Use of this natural topical product for the treatment of various medical conditions was discovered in 1935. This drug is effective for the treatment of skin inflammation as well as minor burns. There are no side effects nor are there are any known drug interactions. Some patients use it for RSD/CRPS pain.

Capsaicin is a drug that has been extensively studied in both the clinical and laboratory settings. Capsaicin is the active component of chili or red peppers. Capsaicin can be put on your skin over your joints if you have joint pain. The capsaicin first stimulates the small pain-transmitting fibers by depleting them of the neurotransmitter substance P. After the substance P has been depleted, you will have a block of the pain fibers that cause burning pain sensations. Observations in Hispanic individuals demonstrated that they did not have mouth or stomach pain after ingesting red peppers. The reason is the depletion of the substance P in the nerve endings in these areas following continual exposure to red peppers.

Substance P also is present in your joints throughout your body. For this reason, capsaicin can be an effective pain reliever for the treatment of pain associated with osteoarthritis and rheumatoid arthritis. It may take a week for you to feel the pain-relieving effects of capsaicin. As substance P is being depleted from your nerve endings, you nerve endings still manufacture substance P. As a result, it will take several days to deplete enough of the substance P to provide you with pain relief. Once you discontinue use of this cream, your nerves will replenish substance P and your pain may return.

Some studies have shown that if you have a neuropathy related to your diabetes you could have significant pain relief with topical capsaicin. Some pain-medicine physicians have used topical capsaicin to relieve the pain associated with shingles. You may have a brief burning sensation following the use of capsaicin. You should be warned to avoid contact with your eyes and genital areas. It is recommended that you use rubber gloves when applying the capsaicin cream. You should use the capsaicin cream no more than three times a day. Various concentrations of capsaicin exist. Begin with a small concentration that contains 0.025 percent capsaicin. You may eventually increase your capsaicin dose to 0.075 percent capsaicin.

Menthol is an oil that is one component of peppermint oil. This oil in a cream base can significantly decrease your pain. When you place a menthol preparation on your skin, the menthol will feel cold to your nerve endings. While you feel the cold, your pain-stimulating nerves will be depressed. Following the initial cool sensation, you will feel a period of warmth. Menthol products can be used for the treatment of pain associated with arthritis, muscle pain, and tendonitis. Application of a menthol-containing cream may be of benefit to you if you suffer from tension headaches. It can be rubbed around the neck muscles just below the skull. It can be an extremely effective method for the treatment of your headaches.

Allergic reactions with menthol have been reported. It is recommended that you test a small amount of menthol on your skin before applying it extensively to assure yourself that you are not allergic it. You should not use the menthol preparation more than three times a day. Do not use a heating pad or a cold pack over the area of your skin where the menthol substance was placed.

Some natural herbs and vegetables can be used as a topical analgesic. One example is an onion. It is reported by some doctors that spreading the juice of a sliced onion over one of your painful areas could reduce your pain. A tincture can be made by putting 100 grams of minced onions in 30 grams of ethanol for a 70 percent solution. There are no hazards or side effects associated with the topical administration of an onion. However, frequent contact with the onion over time could possibly lead to an allergic reaction. The bark of a poplar tree also can be used for relieving your pain. The bark can be used for control of your pain over your joints or nerves or if you have rheumatoid arthritis. You should not use the bark if you are allergic to aspirin. When externally applied using the poplar bark and leaves, you should use no more than five grams of the drug per day.

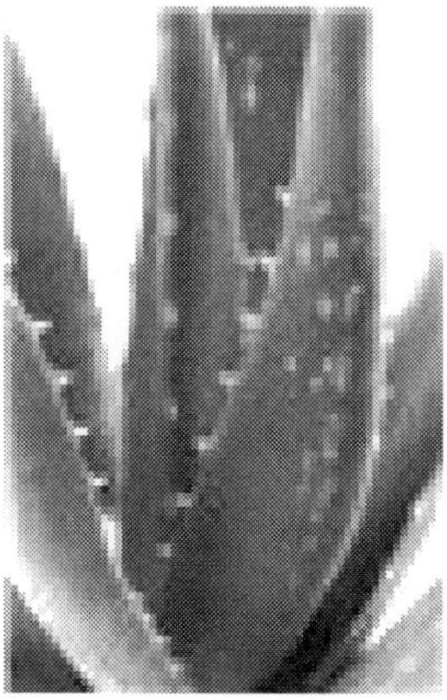

Figure 1. Some plant extracts may be helpful in controlling RSD/CRPS pain.

Another topical medication used to prevent pain is EMLA cream. It is used as a numbing agent more than it is used for reducing pain. This is a cream consisting of lidocaine and prilocaine, which are both numbing agents. This local anesthetic combination is packaged in tubes. There also is an EMLA cellulose disc that can be applied over your painful area. The purpose of this medication is to provide pain relief over the area of the skin. It is used in children to reduce the pain of starting intravenous lines. Some pain-management doctors advocate its use to decrease the pain associated with reflex sympathetic dystrophy or the pain associated with shingles. This cream should be placed on an intact skin area. The EMLA cream should be applied under a bandage for at least 60 minutes to provide relief over the painful area of your skin. This cream is not recommended if you have an allergy to lidocaine or prilocaine. If you have the blood disorder methemoglobinemia, you should not use this cream. You should not exceed the recommended dose prescribed by your physician.

The problem with this cream as opposed to the Lidoderm patches is that it does provide pain relief for your skin. This means that you have a block of all sensation in the skin treated with this cream. You should avoid causing any trauma to the area, including scratching your skin or rubbing or exposing your skin to extreme hot or cold temperatures until you have complete return of sensation to your skin. It is recommended that you not use this medication if you are taking heart medication. The local anesthetics in this cream can interact with some heart medicines.

Another analgesic cream that is available is a combination of methyl salicylate and menthol. This is a cream that is effective for the temporary relief of arthritis and pain in your muscles. You should not use this medicine if your skin is sensitive to the oil of wintergreen. You should apply this cream around the sore areas on your body. You should not apply this cream more than three times a day. Do not place this cream over areas of the skin that are broken

Steroid creams are sometimes used for the treatment of joint pain. Topical steroids are anti-inflammatory agents. Pramoxine hydrochloride is a topical anesthetic agent that sometimes is combined with steroids to attempt to manage pain. This cream provides a temporary relief from pain. You should not use this cream if you are allergic to any of the substances in the cream such as the steroid or the pramoxine. If you develop a rash or blistering, you must stop using the cream. You should not use this cream more than three times a day. Furthermore, do not use this steroid preparation for more than five days. Do not reuse this cream until you have discussed the situation with your doctor.

Nonsteroidal anti-inflammatory agents (NSAIDS) that are commonly taken by mouth for the treatment of bone, joint, and muscle pain may be placed into a cream by your pharmacist. For these drugs to give you pain relief, they must penetrate your skin and enter your bloodstream. These creams should not be used more than three times a day. Side effects with the nonsteroidal anti-inflammatory creams are the same as with the NSAIDs taken by mouth. However, the side effects of the topical NSAIDS are less than the oral NSAIDS. The side effects of any NSAID can include stomach upset and allergic reactions. If the dose is high enough, it could affect your liver and kidneys. The Voltaren gel and the Flector patch are two examples of topical NSAIDs. These NSAIDs can be very effective for the management of your pain when applied over your skin. The use of a ketoprofen gel and a diclofenac gel, both NSAIDs, were compared at painful sites in a four-week study. The ketoprofen gel gave positive results for the treatment of knee pain and was shown to be better at relieving pain than the diclofenac gel. If you have joint pain, you may want to discuss these facts with your pain-medicine doctor or orthopedic doctor. Aspirin creams also may provide you with some pain relief when applied over your painful joints or muscles.

New research is being done into the topical administration of amitriptyline and ketamine. Ketamine is a potent analgesic that can cause you to hallucinate if the dose is too high. A study in animals has used both of these agents together to treat pain in the laboratory setting.

Amitriptyline, which is an antidepressant, has recently been shown to have pain-relieving properties when applied topically. Amitriptyline cream may be advantageous if you do not want to take amitriptyline pills by mouth. The amitriptyline cream will not help you if you are suffering from significant depression, but can be helpful in decreasing your pain. Some people complain of being tired while taking amitriptyline. However, amitriptyline can contribute to pain relief in fibromyalgia and the topical application may be a way of avoiding significant side effects that can be associated with oral use. There is ongoing research in this area. You may want to keep informed of the research on both of these drugs through the National Library of Medicine website at www.nlm.nih.gov.

Another popular patch that is readily available by prescription from your pain-management doctor is the lidocaine-containing patch called Lidoderm. The Lidoderm transdermal drug-delivery system exerts a significant amount of its pain-relieving effects by releasing a small amount of lidocaine into your bloodstream. There also is an effect on the nerves under your skin that are transmitting pain. The Lidoderm patch contains 5 percent lidocaine. The lidocaine essentially does not reach your bloodstream like fentanyl does in the fentanyl patch delivery system. The lidocaine penetrates your skin just enough to reach the nerve endings that are transmitting your pain. As a result, there are minimal side effects from the use of this patch other than from the adhesive layer of the patch. The amount of the lidocaine that is absorbed from the Lidoderm is related to the length of application over your skin. The patch should be used for 12 hours over your painful area and then removed for 12 hours. If an irritation or a burning sensation occurs around the adhesive aspect of the patch, you should discontinue use of the patch. None of the patches mentioned in this chapter should ever be reused.

The Lidoderm patch has a polyester felt backing covered with a polyethylene film release liner. Prior to applying the patch on your skin, the release liner must be removed. Be aware that the patch does contain methylparaben, which is found in many suntan lotions. Do not use the Lidoderm patch if you have allergies to any suntan lotions that contain this chemical.

Clonidine is another transdermal medication. This patch is applied weekly to an area of your skin. The clonidine patch inhibits the release of norepinephrine, which is a RSD/CRPS pain transmitter. The clonidine patch also is used for the treatment of hypertension. If you have neuropathic (nerve injury) pain or reflex sympathetic dystrophy, the clonidine patch may provide you with significant pain relief. It can significantly decrease the burning component of your pain.

You can conclude from this chapter that some topical drugs may be effective for control of your RSD/CRPS pain.

19. Complimentary Medications

"Conventional medicine" is considered to be practiced by individuals who have a medical doctor degree (M.D.) or a doctor of osteopathy degree (D.O.). Conventional medicine also includes methods practiced by allied health-care professionals such as physical therapists, occupational therapists, psychologists, and registered nurses. Other terms for conventional medicine include allopathy, mainstream medicine, and orthodox medicine. In contrast, complementary and alternative medicine are referred to as unconventional or nonconventional medicine as well as unproven health care. Practitioners of alternative medicine hold to the theory that germs can cause illness only if there is an imbalance in various body systems allowing the germs to thrive. They believe that the body's internal environment is healthy and must be kept healthy, and that everyday exposure to germs does not result in illness.

The following is a definition for alternative medicine specialties by the National Center for Complementary and Alternative Medicine. "Complementary and alternative medicines are practices and products that are not currently considered to be part of conventional medicine." Complementary and alternative medicine practices change and update continually. Those therapies that have been thoroughly investigated and that are proven to be safe and effective eventually do become adopted into the conventional health-care system.

Complementary and alternative medicines, unlike many conventional medicine therapies, are designed to help you develop control over your overall health. If you are going to use any of these methods, you are encouraged to learn the side effects of some of these medications as well as learn about drug interactions with medications that you currently may be taking. Inasmuch, do not be afraid to tell your physician what complementary medicines you are taking. Complementary and alternative medicine practices may help you control RSD pain on occasion and should be considered as a form of treatment as an alternative to narcotic medications.

The purpose of this chapter is not to condemn or advocate the utilization of nonconventional medicine practices and substances but to educate you that you can have some control over your overall health as well as control over your pain. Medical professionals are beginning to recognize the benefits of alternative medicine. As an example, the National Institute of Health Office of Alternative Medicine was established in 1992. In addition, there has been a significant increase in professional interest in the area of alternative medicine. Right now, about 30 medical schools are currently offering at least one elective course on alternative medical therapies. The attitudes of medical school faculty toward the use of complementary medicine practices are important.

Here are some other ways that alternative medicine is gaining acceptance: Some health plans have announced their intention to incorporate payment for some alternative medicine practices into their insurance coverage. Some managed care corporations have revealed their intentions to include alternative medicine practices for payment. Some state governments are considering legislation pertaining to the practice of alternative medicine by health-care professionals. If you are going to use a natural substance or therapy, you are responsible for your own care. You must not self-diagnose. You must discuss your symptoms of pain with your physician before taking any nutritional supplement. There are risks and benefits that you should be aware of when using alternative medications and therapies to manage your pain. In addition, the alternative medications you take could react with the prescription medications your doctor has given you and cause you even more problems.

If in doubt, consult the Physician's Drug Reference for herbal medicines. This will advise you about safe doses and any precautions and drug interactions that you may need to be aware of. There was a study published previously in the New England Journal of Medicine in 1993 that was a survey of individuals. More than 30 percent of those surveyed chose alternative medicine over conventional medicine methods to prevent and treat disease .In 1994, Congress passed the Dietary Supplement Health and Education Act. In passing this act, Congress recognized that many individuals believed that dietary supplements offered health benefits. The bill gave dietary supplement manufacturers freedom to produce more products and to provide information about their products' health benefits.

The Food and Drug Administration (FDA), on the other hand, is responsible for overseeing any claims by the dietary supplement manufacturers to the truthfulness of these claims. The Federal Trade Commission regulates the advertising of all of the dietary supplements. You should be aware that the quality control standards for natural substances are a problem within this industry. Some of the manufacturers of these products will not have the amount of substance in the natural medication as stated on the container label. You must do your own research to determine whether the natural substance that you are taking has an accurate dosage as stated on the container label for the product. Remember the drug can be actually less than what the label states. A good rule of thumb for you to consider is that if one product is much cheaper than an identical product, you may want to consider purchasing the more expensive product. The reason for this is that companies that follow appropriate standards usually have their own quality-control systems in effect. As a result, they will have a higher overhead and will have to charge more for the natural medication.

It should be emphasized that the FDA has no control over alternative substances that are categorized as "supplements," and that this has huge quality implications when these agents are compared with conventional drugs. In an Atlanta medical school, 200 full and part-time medical school faculty were given a survey concerning alternative medicine practices. The 24-item survey was given to each medical school faculty member. Three of the 24 items requested participants to respond to a list of 30 specific alternative medical therapies, which included the following: Whether they saw alternative medicine as a legitimate medical practice. Whether they have had personal experience with alternative medicines and felt that they were effective. Whether they have had training in alternative medicine science

Eighty-five of the responders said they have had training in at least one alternative medical therapy. Fifty-seven percent of the responders said they had training in five or more alternative medicine therapies. More than 80 percent had a personal experience with at least one alternative medical therapy and close to 50 percent of the responders reported personal experience with five or more different alternative medical therapies. Almost 90 percent of these alternative medicine experiences were rated effective. Only 3 percent were rated not effective. Less than 1 percent of the medical school faculty felt that these therapies were potentially harmful. The results of this Atlanta medical school study demonstrated that the medical school faculty had a positive exposure to alternative medical therapies. This study is important because medical school faculty members have the responsibility for the education and training of future physicians.

The NIH does award grants for the study of research in complementary as well as alternative medicines. Clinical trials are being done throughout the United States with respect to complementary and alternative medicines. You may want to participate in one of these trials. Trials with respect to herbal medicines are an important part of the medical research process. The results from clinical trials can define better ways to treat your painful conditions. A clinical trial is a research study in which a therapy is tested on individuals like yourself to ensure that the what is being tested is safe and effective. Always remember that clinical trials have risks. Before participating in a clinical trial, discuss this trial with your primary care physician. To find out about ongoing clinical trials for example, studies on arthritis and neurological disorders such as RSD/CRPS go to www.nccam.nih.gov. You also may want to access the National Library of Medicine online (www.pubmed.com). Complementary medicine on PubMed is available that contains citations to articles on recently published research.

Homeopathic specialists prescribe dilutions of natural substances from plants, minerals, and animals. Homeopathy has been around for more than 200 years. About 500 million people around the world receive homeopathic treatment. The World Health Organization has recommended that homeopathy is a system of traditional medicine that should be integrated with conventional medicine, which is considered the traditional approach to medicine. It is important to know that the U.S. Food and Drug Administration recognizes homeopathic remedies as official drugs and regulates their manufacture. This is unlike the herbs used for medicinal use. Homeopathy qualities of medicine are used frequently by conventional physicians in Europe. In Britain, homeopathy is a part of the national health system.

The basic principles of homeopathy are that a disease can be destroyed and removed by a type of medicine that is able to produce the disease in humans. In other words, a substance that in large doses would produce symptoms of a disease can be used in very minute doses to cure it. In conventional medicine, this is called the theory of antibiotics. Homeopathic practitioners adhere to the fact that the more a substance is diluted, the more potent it is. In conventional medicine, it is believed that a higher dose of the medicine will lead to a greater effect.

The purpose of diluting out substances in homeopathic medicine is to avoid side effects. Homeopathic practitioners adhere to the fact that illness is different for every person. Homeopathic treatments are unique for each patient. Homeopathic medicine emphasizes that patients are individuals and have individual signs and symptoms of an illness and should be treated only on an individual basis. The entire individual is treated, which includes the physical, psychological and spiritual portions of each person.

Naturopathic medicine treats disease by using your body's natural ability to heal itself. Naturopathic practitioners invoke healing processes by using a variety of treatment options based on your particular needs. In naturopathic medicine, disease symptoms are a sign of your body's attempt to heal itself naturally. Naturopathic medicine gets its data from Chinese, Native American, and Greek cultures. Naturopaths recommend healing of the person and not the disease. Naturopathic medicinal treatments will include doses of natural substances that are much higher than those used by practitioners of homeopathic medicine.

Even though your primary care physician may not "believe" in complementary and alternative medications, you should not be afraid to approach your doctor with the fact that you are taking herbal medications. This is important not only because of possible drug interactions, but because some substances such as garlic and gingko can decrease your blood's ability to form a blood clot normally. This could result in excessive bleeding. It is extremely important if you are about to have a surgical procedure that you let your surgeon know you are taking an herb that can thin your blood. You surgery may need to be delayed until your blood's ability to form a normal clot has been restored.

Be aware that when you are using alternative medicines that these medicines are not strictly controlled with respect to dosage and the amount of drug in a pill, capsule, or tea. All plants have different amounts of substances in them. A true dose of a medication is unknown in many instances. You should look carefully at the label before taking one of these substances and not take more than the label recommends. The overall drug interactions of herbal substances have not been established because they are not required to be strictly studied by the FDA. To best choose a natural product to decrease your pain, you should know which chemicals in the body produce pain.

With this knowledge, you can pick the analgesic best suited to relieve your pain. If you have joint pain, for instance, you will want to use an alternative medicine that has anti-inflammatory properties. If you are injured or have inflammation, your body makes a variety of chemicals that transmit pain impulses to a pain-processing center in your brain. These chemicals include the prostaglandins, cytokines, substance P, glutamic acid, and nitric oxide. Nitric oxide is a gas that is a pain chemical transmitter in your nervous system. This should not be confused with nitrous oxide, which is used for pain control in dental procedures.

The following remedies are anti-inflammatory substances that you may want to use as a prostaglandin inhibitor to relieve your pain: Tumeric has anti-inflammatory and antioxidant effects and has been shown to inhibit prostaglandin formation. This drug should not be used if you have gallbladder disease. No significant health risks or side effects with use of this drug have been reported to date. The average dose is 3 grams of tumeric per day. This dose can be divided up into 1-gram doses and be taken 3 times per day with meals. For example, you may take 1 milligram with each meal for a total dose of 3 grams.

Ginseng has anti-inflammatory effects and is used in homeopathic medicine for the treatment of rheumatoid arthritis. You should not use this medicine if you have hypertension. Do not use ginseng with caffeine. Exercise caution if you use ginseng along with any antidiabetic medicine or insulin. You should not use ginseng with MAOI inhibitors, which are used to decrease your blood pressure. Do not use ginseng in combination with diuretics. Side effects include sleep deprivation, nosebleeds, headaches, nervousness, and vomiting. The average daily dose of this root is 1 to 2 grams. Do not take more than 2 grams per day. The 2 grams can be divided up and taken 3 times a day.

Resveratrol is an antioxidant and a COX-2 inhibitor that some believe prevents heart disease and cancer. It is largely found in the skin of red grapes. Therefore, many people obtain resveratol by drinking red wine. This substance can prevent clot formation, whereas the conventional COX-2 inhibitors do not prevent clot formation. The usual dose is no more than 600 mmg per day. There are no known side effects or drug interactions for resveratrol itself.

Fish oils contain the omega-3 fatty acids and can decrease prostaglandins. Fish oils are used for the treatment of rheumatoid arthritis. You also may use fish oils for the control of joint pain. The most common side effect that you may experience with fish oil supplementation is mild stomach upset. The fish oils can decrease your blood's ability to clot. If you are taking blood-thinning drugs, you should not take fish oils, because it will give you an increased risk of bleeding. You may take up to -10 grams of fish oil per day.

N-acetylcysteine is an amino acid produced by your body that will decrease prostaglandin N-acetylcysteine formation. It can help prevent some diseases and boost your immune system. You should not take this drug if you are taking carbamazepine (Tegretol). Side effects include headaches, nausea, vomiting, and stomach upset. The recommended dose is 200 milligrams 3 times a day.

Cayenne is an anti-inflammatory medication that is helpful for the treatment of muscle pain and arthritis. This drug may be helpful for inhibiting the release of substance P as well. Cayenne side effects include diarrhea and intestinal colic. It can decrease your body's ability to form a normal blood clot. It also can reduce the effects of aspirin, so you should be aware of this fact if you are taking aspirin as a blood thinner. High doses of cayenne over a prolonged time can cause kidney and liver damage. You should not use this drug for more than two days in a row. After two weeks you may use it again for two days. The daily dose of cayenne should not exceed 10 grams.

Ipriflavone can be used as a prostaglandin inhibitor. Women also use it to decrease the incidence of osteoporosis. This medicine can actually stop bone loss. It can decrease the risk of fractures in bone pain in females. This drug, like the other drugs that are prostaglandin inhibitors, can increase the blood-thinning activity of other drugs that you may be taking, such as Coumadin. It also can increase the effects of some asthma drugs such as theophylline, so avoid taking ipriflavone if you are using such medications. Side effects are mostly stomach upset. The average dose is 200 milligrams 3 times a day.

Procyanidolic oligomers are natural substances extracted from grape seeds. They are useful for their antioxidant effects. They can decrease arthritis pain. However, another important effect of this medicine is that it can decrease the effects of nitric oxide. Nitric oxide is released from cells in your bloodstream. Nitric acid essentially exists in a gas form to transmit pain impulses. One side effect of this medicine that has been reported is that it increased the effects of dextroamphetamine (Dexedrine) in a child who had an attention deficit disorder. There are no significant side effects associated with this drug. The daily dose of this drug ranges from 150 to 300 milligrams per day.

Cytokine inhibitors include the fish oils, as previously mentioned. Cytokines are chemicals produced in your bloodstream that enhance pain impulses. They contribute to the formation of substances that can destroy your joint linings if you have rheumatoid arthritis. Substance P inhibitors include cayenne and ginseng. Substance P is a neurotransmitter chemical that can be associated with nerve pain, such as shingles. If you have shingles, you may want to consider using a substance P inhibitor.

Histamine also can provide you with pain relief. Histamine released from certain cells in your body can cause you to develop a rash, a headache, and itching all over your body. However, in extremely small doses, histamine may relieve your pain. There have not been any placebo-controlled studies to date that compare a histamine cream to a placebo cream. However, one animal study did conclude that morphine may exert its pain-relieving effect in the brain and spinal cord by releasing histamine into the central nervous system.

Hydroxytryptophan is an amino acid that naturally occurs in your body. It has been found to significantly decrease substance P formation. Because substance P may be involved in fibromyalgia, this medicine can improve your fibromyalgia pain. It also may helpful for the treatment of headaches, shingles, and neuropathic pain entities such as carpal tunnel syndrome.

Nausea is a common side effect of this drug. You also may experience drowsiness, dry mouth, and stomach pain. In 1989, some people taking this drug developed joint pain, high fever, weakness in their arms and legs, and had shortness of breath.

The Center for Disease Control concluded that the drug came from a Japanese manufacturer and was contaminated. Drug interactions reveal severe effects if a person is taking an antidepressant medicine from their doctor. You should not take this drug if you have Parkinson's disease and are not taking the drug Sinemet. Do not use this drug if you have scleroderma. This drug also may interfere with the effects of drugs that you may be taking for migraine headaches. Adults should take no more than 50 milligrams 3 times a day.

Cannabinoids are another natural substance for the control of pain. State legislation throughout the United States will eventually make a decision on the use of cannabinoids for medical purposes. Marijuana has been used since antiquity. In 1942, marijuana was reported to be a dangerous, harmful, and addictive drug. In 1970, marijuana was classified as a highly addictive drug with no accepted medical use. However, in 1996, voters in Arizona and California passed referenda to legalize marijuana for medicinal use. To date, doctors are prohibited from prescribing marijuana for medical conditions. There has been a recent discovery of two cannabinoid receptors, CB-1 and CB-2. Now the scientific medical community is interested in this substance.

Cannabinoids are now reported to have therapeutic value as pain relievers. This means that marijuana could help you with your pain in many situations. There have not been any controlled clinical trials for the use of this drug. Cannabinoids do exhibit some anti-inflammatory properties. However, they are no more effective than the current anti-inflammatory medications available. If you suffer from pain involving your nerves, such as shingles or reflex sympathetic dystrophy, you may be able to note some pain relief with the use of marijuana. To date the safety and efficacy of marijuana has not been found. In 1997, the American Medical Association House of Delegates recommended adequately designed controlled studies with respect to pain as well as other illnesses.

Acupuncturists practice alternative medicine methods. Acupuncture is used in traditional Chinese medicine. It involves inserting fine needles into the body at specific points that have been found to be effective in the treatment of specific health problems. The purpose of acupuncture is to balance the body's flow of energies. Acupuncture can relieve pain, and those who perform acupuncture say it is able to restore health. Sometimes acupuncturists will burn herbs around a specific acupressure point for added relief.

Chiropractic medicine has been around since 1895. It is the second largest health profession in the world and one of the fastest growing. Chiropractors are aware of the possible dangers posed by conventional medical procedures. Chiropractors have found the nonmedical approach to body ailments that uses the body's own healing abilities to restore health. Chiropractic medicine emphasizes individual well-being, including having a healthful diet and using natural medicines. Chiropractic therapy can be extremely effective in the management of painful conditions of the spine. Chiropractors do not prescribe conventional medicines, but do recommend natural substances that can promote healing of the body and prevent illnesses.

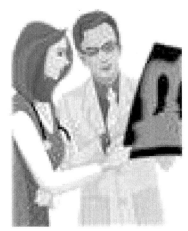

Figure 1. Your chiropractor will review your X rays and do a thorough physical examination before initiating treatment.

In summary, although the symptoms may be devastating and the medical prognosis poor at best, there are very specific chiropractic neurological protocols that can be followed to afford these patients some relief. Isolation of the initial nociception must be accomplished first and foremost, to assure that we eliminate any further nociceptive barrage into the nervous system and IML. If it is a chronic patient, many times the initial causative factor has long since healed and may not even be associated with the present condition. The next step to address by chiropractic therapy is to promote large-diameter afferent neuronal barrage into the apical internuncial pool through some stimulus of the system. This could be accomplished by any of the means mentioned previously, with the possibilities of treatment too numerous to address specifically in this chapter. The final factor to address is treatment of the opposite side of pain, to promote thalamic-hypothalamic-reticulo-spinal pathways and inhibit nociception supraseg-mentally. In my experience, when all of these factors are brought into play efficaciously, there are positive and long-standing results that cannot be underestimated in the eyes of a suffering patient.

RSD/CRPS symptoms may be managed with a combination of painkillers and cold-laser treatment; cold-laser treatment is used to treat both chronic and acute pain, and may be an effective mode of therapy for RSD sufferers. Cold-laser therapy does not emit any heat, but does emit low-power light waves over the treatment area to reduce inflammation. Cold-laser therapy uses a combination of electrical stimulation and cold-laser beams to increase serotonin levels in the body and allow the body to heal naturally. Cold-laser therapy has been proven effective for the treatment of chronic and acute pain in more than 100 successful randomized double-blind clinical trials. Cold-laser therapy for RSD works by emitting electromagnetic energy directly into the skin tissues. These energy waves are absorbed by the mitochondria in the cell, and are converted to chemical energy. This stimulates the cells at a deep level and encourages healing, thereby reducing the sensation of pain, and triggering the natural healing process.

Cold-laser therapy for RSD sufferers can be used on nearly any area of the body, including the knees, elbows, upper back, neck, shoulders and other inflamed joints. Some of the key benefits of cold-laser therapy for RSD sufferers are: reduction of pain without medication, non-invasive treatment, improved rate of tissue repair for natural healing, enhanced sense of well-being, no medication needed to complement treatment, reduction of skin sensitivity in the treated area and progressive results.

It can be concluded that complimentary medicine can be an adjunct to conventional medicine for the treatment of RSD/CRPS.

20. Behavioral Therapy

Patients with RSD/CRPS can exhibit various types of pain behaviors. In 1976, Fordyce suggested that pain behavior is a learned response that can be modified. If a patient receives extra attention from a spouse or family members, the pain behavior is "reinforced." This is an example of pain causing a benefit or a "positive reinforcement." On the other hand, if an individual loses work and income because of pain, pain intensity usually decreases, allowing the individual to return to work. This is an example of "negative reinforcement." Both the patient and the doctor need to identify situations that reinforce pain behavior.

Patients can use a pain diary to help identify what behavior signals pain, and a family conference may help to identify the positive reinforcements (rewards) of pain, such as a doting spouse, being excused from household chores, and so on. Some people appreciate extra attention given them by family members, attention that perhaps was not available before the painful condition. Others use pain to avoid psychologically painful situations, such as workplace problems with co-workers or a supervisor, and use it to avoid going to work and dealing with colleagues. People may also use pain to avoid social or family gatherings.

When doctors fail to relieve pain, patients may find that a consultation with a behavioral medicine specialist such as a psychologist or psychiatrist may prove helpful. If pain provides a way to escape difficult psychological situations, this should be addressed. Most people with pain respond to routine treatments, such as oral medication and nerve injections of anti-inflammatory drugs (corticosteroids, for instance) as well as physical or manipulative therapy. When an individual fails to respond to these methods, psychological intervention is necessary.

Pain patient behaviors that should be closely watched include frequently talking about pain, moaning, and frequently going to doctors and refusing to work. Doctors should observe and note blatant pain manifestations. Pain behavior is influenced by environmental consequences. Suffering is the conceptual component of pain that denotes a persistent negative affect. Suffering is composed of depression, fear, and isolation.

The concept of pain is complex. Dr. Gerald Aronoff, a noted psychiatrist with a specialty in pain medicine, has reported that patients with chronic pain share many of the following characteristics: preoccupation with pain, strong dependency needs, feelings of isolation, an inability to attend to self needs, and an inability to appropriately deal with repressed anger and hostility. Pain and disability can cause dependency upon others to assist in activities of daily living, such a cooking, cleaning, laundry, and so on. Many chronic pain patients have suffered emotionally traumatic childhoods; a history of this trauma should be sought by the doctors caring for these patients. Pain may significantly increase when there is low self-esteem. Emotional disorders can also be associated with chronic pain, including somataform disorders, somatization disorders, conversion disorders, psychogenic pain disorders, and hypochondriasis. These emotional disorders will affect a patient's response to a chronic pain syndrome.

In a somataform disorder, physical symptoms are compatible with a physical disorder, but there is no evidence of any clear psychiatric or physical problem. These patients overanalyze their bodies and have a tendency to look for abnormal symptoms. A somatization disorder is a chronic disorder that usually begins before age 30 and primarily affects women. With it, an individual complains of many symptoms but has few physical findings to confirm their complaints. These individuals consult many doctors to validate their symptoms and may even consent to multiple injections by a pain-management doctor or even a surgical procedure for the treatment of pain.

A conversion disorder results from an emotional conflict unrelated to bodily disease but resulting in loss of function of a part of the body. An example is losing the use of a hand without an obvious physical problem or injury. These individuals exaggerate the magnitude of their complaints. Psychogenic pain disorders are complaints of pain without adequate physical findings. These individuals exhibit neurotic behavior. Neurotic behavior is a behavior that you realize is abnormal such as anxiety. Individuals seeking financial compensation may exhibit psychogenic pain disorders. Hypochondriasis is a disturbance that involves an unrealistic interpretation of physical disease. These individuals have a preoccupation with the belief that they have a serious disease and are preoccupied with their physical symptoms.

Malingering is uncommon but implies a conscious fabrication of an illness for personal gain. These individuals are often seeking financial compensation or may be seeking narcotic analgesic drugs such as morphine or Dilaudid. The pain-prone patient is often an individual who had a traumatic childhood, perhaps with a history of physical and/or emotional abuse or a history of chronic pain or disability. Individuals who feel unloved are prone to use pain to meet ungratified needs. These individuals frequently try to manipulate others and have a tendency to burden their families.

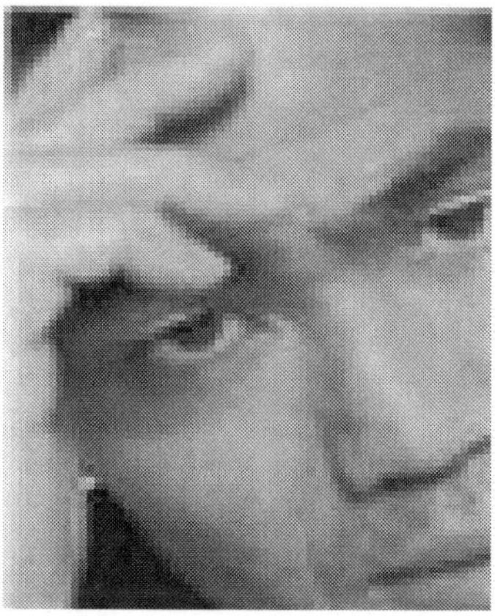

Figure 1. RSD/CRPS pain patients with psychological illnesses can be a burden to those who associate with them.

Various psychological tests are available to evaluate pain patients. A common test is the Minnesota Multiphase Personality Inventory Test (MMPI), which evaluates multiple dimensions of a pain patient. The Beck Depression Scale can be used to assess depression. The MMPI, consisting of 566 questions, is widely used by psychologists working with pain patients, but cannot consistently distinguish between psychogenic and tissue damage pain. However, people with high hypochondriasis and hysteria scores and lower depression scores may have a physical basis for their pain, rather than a conversion reaction. The MMPI test also proves useful in assessing emotional disorders that occur secondary to a pain experience and personality factors that could affect an individual's response to pain treatment.

A problem with labeling pain as psychogenic is the assumption that the actual cause of the affected patient's pain is unknown. This assumption may be false, because the physical reason for many pain syndromes may be unclear or unknown. This is a problem in workman's compensation or bodily injury cases. If, following an examination, a doctor paid by an insurance company cannot find a reason for a claimant's pain, the patient is often labeled as a malingerer, which unfortunately ruins the patient's credibility with a judge or jury. Remember, however, that the diagnosis of psychogenic pain is a diagnosis only of exclusion. That is, a diagnosis made by excluding the diseases to which only some of your symptoms may belong, leaving one disease as the most likely diagnosis, although no conclusive tests or findings establish that diagnosis for certain.

Most pain doctors want to minimize the use of drugs and medicines. No medicine is without potential dangerous side effects. This is why most pain-management doctors use injection therapy and prescribe physical and/or occupational therapy and make referrals to chiropractors or other nonconventional health-care providers. In the past, the failure of injections or drugs to relieve pain resulted in referral to a psychologist or a psychiatrist for treatment of psychiatric or behavioral problems. Today these specialists are essential to pain management. In fact, a psychiatrist is a medical doctor, and a psychologist has a Ph.D. Not only can psychiatrists prescribe medications for pain, they also attend to mental and emotional conditions that may be contributing to pain. (A psychologist cannot prescribe medication.)

Psychological assessments and treatment are now part of the total approach to managing those experiencing chronic pain. Psychologists can teach relaxation techniques and biofeedback and use hypnosis to decrease pain, complementing physical therapy, pharmacological therapy, and injections. Therefore, you should not feel offended if your pain-management doctor wants to send you to a psychologist. Instead, welcome this method and be aware that the psychologist will help you take control of your own pain. Remember that pain medicine is not a "cookbook" approach to diagnosing and treating pain. A multidisciplinary approach, one that treats the whole patient, is the proper way to manage your pain.

People's expectations when seeing a pain doctor or receiving medications, nerve injections, and psychological therapy will also affect their pain responses. Those who do not expect relief, on the other hand, will probably not experience pain relief. For this reason, each individual has control of his or her painful situation. You can observe the pain patterns of animals to realize that in humans there must be a strong psychological component to a chronic pain syndrome. For example, a dog or cat can be struck by an automobile and sustain significant trauma. In most instances, however, the animal is back functioning within a short time. An animal has no secondary gain issues and does not anticipate having significant monetary compensation for an injury caused by a careless driver. However, humans can have prolonged pain following an accident only to have the pain relieved following a large jury settlement. This observation is referred to as the "green poltice" treatment.

Methods used by psychologists for the management of pain include relaxation and biofeedback training. These methods are used to treat both acute and chronic pain syndromes. Relaxation is also frequently used to control pain associated with labor contractions. Used properly, relaxation can also decrease the body's metabolic activity and preserve energy. Learning to manage pain through relaxation methods enables people to consciously control pain and become proactive in their own pain management.

Biofeedback is another method of treatment frequently used by psychologists to manage pain. An electromyogram, which measures muscle contractions in different parts of the body, can be used for biofeedback training and pain evaluations. Other measurements include skin temperature and brainwave forms. When muscles are tense, skin temperature is less than in surrounding tissues because of a decrease in blood flow. Biofeedback techniques can increase blood flow to muscles and skin and increase your temperature. This can be used in combination with relaxation training to manage pain; both techniques are more commonly used by women than by men. Biofeedback has been used to treat many chronic pain syndromes, including muscle-tension headaches. People with migraine headaches, phantom limb pain, and reflex sympathetic dystrophy can also respond to biofeedback training.

Relaxation treatment has also been shown to be effective for the management of lower back pain. Most back pain is caused by sustained muscle tension. Relaxation training relaxes muscles and increases blood flow and oxygen delivery while removing excessive buildup in muscles of lactic acid. Be aware, however, that muscle relaxation is not effective in all people. Further, no method described in this book is 100 percent effective for pain control. If you suffer from arthritis of the spine, muscle relaxation will not completely relieve your arthritic pain. Biofeedback has also been shown to be helpful in the management of back pain, especially if related to increased muscle tension. If you suffer from TMJ (temporomandibular joint pain), relaxation techniques and/or biofeedback may also provide you with significant pain relief. Hypnosis is another tool used by psychologists to relieve pain. Hypnosis has a long history of use in various pain syndromes. Hypnosis reduces awareness of painful stimuli by providing suggestions or images that divert attention away from painful stimuli. Hypnosis is a state of consciousness that differs from the normal waking state and is characterized by a significant response to suggestions, although not everyone responds to hypnotic therapy.

Hypnosis can decrease or inhibit pain impulses to the brain's pain center as well as pain impulses in the spinal cord. Hypnosis can create the expectation of pain reduction. Hypnosis has been used for the management of cancer pain and postoperative pain. Imagery is an important component of hypnosis. Hypnosis causes a deeply relaxed state, diverting attention from pain. When you have pain, if you visualize the pain as a bright red color, you can use imagery to lighten the red to a pink color, which is analogous to a reduction in your pain. If you have burning pain over your skin from shingles, you may imagine cool water and ice being placed over your burning skin. These suggestions and images may prove useful to reduce pain. Although hypnosis is used to reduce pain, it is difficult to completely eliminate it. However, it can decrease pain to a tolerable state.

A psychologist also can help you manage pain through "cognitive-behavioral management" of pain. Cognitive processes are those means by which we become aware of situations. These processes include reasoning and decision making. Behavior is your response to a stimulus. In doing this type of psychological pain relief, your psychologist will analyze your thoughts and feelings as well as your beliefs and what behavior response you use on a painful stimulus. Your psychologist will teach you relaxation as well as what you can do if you have a relapse of your pain syndrome. Your psychologist will help you take control over any abnormal thoughts or feelings. Your psychologist can train you to change your ways of thinking and alter your feelings and behaviors in a manner that can leave you with positive thoughts and subsequently help you relax and control your chronic pain.

Your psychologist will discuss with you concerns that you may have with respect to the health-care system and analyze your patterns of medication use. Your psychologist will evaluate the role of family members and how they can help you manage your pain. You will be taught that negative thoughts can occur, and the occurrence of some negative thoughts is normal. However, when they do occur you are to use those thoughts as reminders to initiate coping skills taught to you by your psychologist. Be aware by now that psychologists not only do tests to assess your levels of depression and anxiety and so forth, they also have treatment methods that are noninvasive and do not involve the administration of drugs. Psychiatrists can also provide you with counseling and in many instances recommend counseling over medications. It is your choice as to which of these methods could work best for you with respect to your pain management.

21. Physical/Occupational Therapy

Physical and/or occupational therapy can be important for the management of RSD/CRPS pain. Physical therapy is an important modality that can be used to help manage your pain. Physical therapists, sometimes referred to as simply PTs, These individuals are healthcare professionals who diagnose and treat individuals of all ages, from newborns to the very oldest, who have medical problems or other health-related conditions, illnesses, or injuries that limits their abilities to move and perform functional activities as well as they would like in their daily lives.

Occupational therapists help patients improve their ability to perform tasks in living and working environments. They work with individuals who suffer from a mentally, physically, developmentally, or emotionally disabling condition. Occupational therapists use treatments to develop, recover, or maintain the daily living and work skills of their patients. The therapist helps clients not only to improve their basic motor functions and reasoning abilities, but also to compensate for permanent loss of function. The goal is to help clients have independent, productive, and satisfying lives. A therapist will rehabilitate you following an injury.

Your physical/occupational therapist will decide which treatment is best for you based on your overall health after an evaluation. Your physical/occupational therapist will emphasize to you that you yourself are a major component in your rehabilitation and in the management of your chronic pain. Your physical/occupational therapist also will train you to avoid future re-injury and/or a recurrence of your pain problems. Not only is a physical/occupational therapy evaluation a planned treatment course for your pain, you also will receive an education on future injury prevention. If you were injured in your workplace, your physical therapist will tell you how to avoid further injury in that environment.

You also may be placed in a work-hardening program to enable you to become maximally conditioned for your occupation. This program duplicates your regular work duties and helps increase your muscle strength and endurance so that you can return safely back to work, hopefully without further injury.

Your therapist will attempt to get you back to normal daily activity as soon as possible in a safe manner. You do not want to return to activity too soon following the onset of sudden pain because you could re-injure yourself or cause yourself a worse injury. When you see your physical therapist on your first visit, you should expect the therapist to obtain a detailed medical history from you. To provide you adequate treatment, your therapist will want to know your complete medical history as well as your pain history. The history that you tell your therapist will give the therapist important information about your pain syndrome, your prognosis, and the appropriate time that you will need to be under the physical therapist's treatments.

Your therapist also will assess your behavioral response to your pain associated with your injury if you were injured in an accident or at work. If your pain has moved or spread since you first noticed it, be sure to tell your therapist. This information is important because RSD/CRPS can spread to other extremities. If your pain is worse in the morning and becomes progressively better during the day, this may be an indication that you have arthritis. Post traumatic arthritis is not uncommon after an injury to your arm or leg. /occupational Your therapist will need to know this information in order to prescribe the proper treatment for you. Providing a good medical history to your therapist will make it much easier for the therapist to prescribe the proper method of treatment for you.

You should write down pertinent information about yourself prior to your first physical therapy visit. Your therapist will need to know if your pain is in your bones, muscles, nerves, or all of them together. If the pain is in your bones, the pain is usually confined to that particular area. If your pain is in a nerve, the pain will usually go down your arm or leg from where the therapist is pressing on your spine or neck. If your pain is in your muscles, your physical therapist will note increased contractility of the painful muscles. Your therapist will examine the range of motion of your joints.

The color of your skin will be noted by your therapist. Sometimes if you have arthritis, there may be redness about your joints. With RSD/CRPS, you skin may have a bluish tint or be shiny. Your hair pattern in your arms and legs will be evaluated. If you have decreased blood flow with your RSD/CRPS, there may be a loss of hair on your skin. Movements of your joints, neck, and lower back will be done to see how flexible you are. Any movements that are painful will be recorded and then will be addressed during your therapy session. Your therapist will decide whether heat or cold could help you with your range of motion or decrease your muscle spasms, which in turn will help decrease your pain. Your physical therapist's examination will emphasize the joints of your body as well as your muscles. The examination by your therapist may be more thorough than the examination by your doctor with respect to joint movement. On examination, your therapist will try to determine what movements worsen your pain.

Your physical therapist will examine you for paralysis or a loss of your reflexes in your arms and legs. Any shrinkage of the muscle in your arms and legs will be addressed. If you cannot use your arm or leg because of RSD/CRPS, your muscle will decrease in size. For example, if you have decreased muscle size in your thigh, your therapist will target this area to increase strength and muscle mass. Your therapist will, furthermore, examine you for any loss of sensation in your arms and legs. For example, if you have a loss of sensation in your right shoulder, your therapist will be careful not to apply heat on this area for any significant length of time. If you have limited range of motion about your arm or leg, your therapist will work with you to increase your range of motion.

A heating pad could cause a burn on your skin if you are unable to detect the sensation of heat about your shoulder. After your therapist has examined you, the therapist may call your doctor to recommend any further laboratory tests or x-rays. After the history and physical examination has been completed, your physical therapist will determine what is causing your pain problem and will design a treatment program for you based on these findings. You will be treated as a complete individual, and not as just a pain symptom. If your assessment was not done thoroughly, your treatment regimen may not help you with respect to your pain syndrome.

Your therapist may do a muscle and joint stabilization program to increase your strength and flexibility. You, on the other hand, must always feel that you are a main component in your rehabilitation. If your therapist gives you exercises to do at home you follow the instructions on how to do them and do them on the prescribed schedule. Your physical therapist will treat you with exercise and strengthening techniques, but also may complement your therapy with whirlpool baths, paraffin baths, or other methods such as using electrical current. Your occupational therapist will evaluate and treat you with respect to function at home as well as in the workplace. For example if you have RSD/CRPS of your hand, your therapist will teach you how to use the painful hand to eat, dress etc.

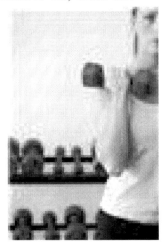

Figure 1. Therapy may include muscle strengthening.

Heat packs can provide you with surface heating, which may reduce the pain in some surface muscles in your back, arms, or legs. Ultrasound is a deep application of heat. This method can relax your deep muscles. Elastic exercise bands and medicine balls may be used to increase your arm and leg strength. The elastic bands can be used to increase your strength, and medicine balls can be used to increase your range of motion and your flexibility as well as your strength. Some physical therapists use traction for the management of your pain. You should avoid ice on the affected extremity that has RSD/CRPS. Cold can decrease blood flow to tour injured skin and muscle which will cause your RSD/CRPS pain to worsen.

Electricity can be used to treat your pain syndrome as well. Over the years, many claims have been made for the therapeutic application of electrical current for the treatment of some pain syndromes. Electrical current is applied to your body by placement of electrodes, which are patches with adhesive that stick to your body. The current is directed over the painful areas of your body. Electrical current can vibrate the molecules of your tissues similar to ultrasound therapy. The vibration produced by friction between the molecules of your tissues will increase your tissue temperature. As a result, heat is produced. As electrical current passes through your tissue, some nerves are excited while others are not. It has been shown that electricity can stimulate tissue growth and repair such as bone and is sometimes used by orthopedic surgeons to stimulate bone growth following bone surgery.

Sometimes stimulators can be placed following orthopedic surgery to enhance bone growth. Theoretically, the electrical current should speed up your healing time. A popular electrical current emitting device that is used frequently in pain medicine by conventional physicians, chiropractic physicians, and physical therapists is the transcutaneous electrical nerve stimulator (TENS).

A TENS unit applies electrical current to your body through electrodes that are adhered to your body. The TENS unit is used for pain control. The power source is battery operated. TENS unit therapy became popular in the late 1960s and early 1970s. The use of a TENS unit for the treatment of your chronic pain syndrome if you have neck, back, arm, and leg pain is well documented. RSD/CRPS pain can be controlled with a TENS unit. A TENS unit has an amplitude knob that lets your control your pain relief. These TENS units are about the size of a pager. The TENS unit patches can be placed over your muscles or nerves for the management of pain both in your muscles as well as the nerves in your arms and legs.

You can use a TENS unit for the control of your pain long term without any significant side effects. Some people have allergic reactions to the adhesive in the patches. Iontophoresis is another use of an electrical current to drive medications through your skin. Different medications can be applied through your skin to decrease your pain. Not only is electrical current used for pain relief, it can also speed up your tissue healing. Phonophoresis is another device that uses energy to drive medications into your body.

In addition, visiting a physical/occupational therapist is often part of the treatment regimen. To take care of patients suffering from this condition, physical therapists often conduct electrical stimulation. The physical therapist may also perform manual techniques such as massage to decrease the pain associated with RSD/CRPS. In addition, the physical therapist may prescribe desensitization techniques including sanding wood, scrubbing and carrying weights. With early intervention and a commitment to physical therapy, the patient can reduce the pain associated with RSD/CRPS. Physical therapy is primarily used to strengthen muscles (although it can also be helpful for building bone density, improving circulation, improving nerve function and endurance). Physical therapy can be "the cure" for some RSD/CRPS patients while others have no response or negative responses to physical therapy.

Functional limitations should be identified. A therapist should define specific functional goals for treatment related to the affected extremity. All RSD/CRPS treatment programs should include: A progressive active exercise program should include progressive weight bearing for lower extremity RSD/CRPS. Progressive improvement of grip strength, pinch strength, and shoulder range of motion of the upper extremity RSD/CRPS should be addressed as well.

A desensitization program using a rough texture may desensitize your painful nerve endings. For specific RSD / CRPS cases, additional treatment options may be indicated to enhance effectiveness of the above elements. For example, bracing of the affected extremity may be necessary. Excessive exercise and physical therapy that causes fatigue, pain, and distress to any part of the body and may aggravate the inflammation and pain of RSD/CRPS. On the other hand, bed rest and inactivity can worsen the symptoms of RSD/CRPS.

Prolonged bed rest results in aggravation of pain and insomnia in RSD/CRPS patients. The RSD/CRPS patients suffer from severe, chronic insomnia due to the constant allodynic pain as well as due to the aggravation of constriction of blood vessels secondary to inactivity. On the other hand, too much exercise can worsen RSD/CRPS pain. Before choosing a therapist, you should interview your potential therapist. You should ascertain if the therapist has experience in treating CRPS/RSD. Do not be treated by a therapist who has no experience with RSD/CRPS.

In summary physical/occupational therapy can benefit patients suffering from RSD/CRPS. As a result, a patient with RSD/CRPS may not need stelate ganglion or lumbar sympathetic injections, surgical sympathectomy, and numerous oral and topical medications, dorsal column stimulators or morphine pumps, all of which are frequently unsuccessful. You should try the least invasive modalities initially. If you have no results from conservative therapy, then and only then are more invasive modalities recommended.

You should know that pain medicine as an entity is not a recognized medical specialty by the American Board of Medical Specialties but is a sub classification with certification awarded by the American Board of Anesthesiology. An anesthesiologist, physical medicine rehabilitation specialist, neurologist, orthopedic surgeon, or neurosurgeon can all call themselves pain specialists, as can psychiatrists, psychologists, and chiropractors. Alternative medicine specialists such as an acupuncturists can call themselves pain management practitioners as well.

A qualified pain physician will be listed in ABMS.org. Website. On the other hand, some practitioners have completed fellowships in pain medicine. These individuals have had comprehensive training at a medical center. These doctors have had training in reading your MRI, CT scan, and so on and training in how to decide whether a patient needs physical therapy, psychological evaluation, medications, or injections therapies to manage pain. A fellowship-trained individual is one who has had special training in his or her specialty, whether it be anesthesiology, physical medicine, rehabilitation, or neurology. These specialty-trained individuals are equipped with the proper tools to treat you as a whole individual. This is not to say that the other individuals are not doing an adequate job for managing your pain.

Some entities such as reflex sympathetic dystrophy are more complex and require the expertise of someone who has a more in-depth knowledge of your disease. This individual may be affiliated with a university pain-management program. Most anesthesiology departments at university medical centers throughout the country have comprehensive pain-medicine programs. This ensures you that you may be evaluated by a physical therapist, occupational therapist, or psychologist. These types of programs offer you multiple methods. The problem is that some insurance plans advise you to stay away from multidisciplinary pain centers because they can be expensive. If you have been involved in a motor vehicle accident or have sustained a work-related injury, and develop RSD/CRPS your case may end up before a court. When choosing your pain-management practitioner, you may want someone who not only can treat your pain but also who can be an expert witness for you in a court of law. No matter what type of individual you choose to manager your pain, remember that individual is ultimately being paid by you. Even if your insurance company is paying the individual, remember that you or your employer are the one who pays the insurance premiums. Because most chronic pain syndromes require long-term care with a health-care provider, you need to ask the health-care provider for a curriculum vitae.

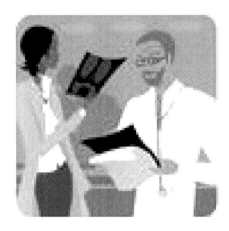

Figure 1. Find a physician who is fellowship trained and board certified in pain management.

A curriculum vitae will show you the qualifications of your potential health-care provider. Most individuals are proud of their accomplishments and will readily furnish you with a resume or a curriculum vitae. If your potential health-care provider does not have this information readily available, you must ascertain the educational background of your health-care provider. You need to know what schools that individual has attended. You may want to know the major areas of study during college and the major areas of study during professional training. Your health-care provider should provide you with any additional courses attended as well as the dates. Some individuals have attended no additional courses in pain management. Some individuals who have previously attended courses have furthermore, not attended additional courses for several years.

However, most state medical boards now require individuals to meet continuing medical education courses to keep their licenses. Other health professions also have this continuing education rule. You need to know if your health-care provider has done a fellowship in pain medicine. This fact is important because remember that anyone can place a shingle outside of his or her office claiming a specialty in pain management.

Most individuals keep a list of the education courses that they have attended in the past 10 years. To be a member of an HMO or certain insurance plans, health-care providers must update their curriculum vitae each year (and submit it to the HMO or insurance company). Your health-care provider should, therefore, have a curriculum vitae that lists what education courses he or she has taken in the past 10 years. You need to know if your health-care provider has been the subject of any disciplinary actions. Sometimes a health-care provider license will not be renewed for various reasons. A common reason is that the individual forgot to pay his or her dues. This is a much different disciplinary action than a disciplinary action for someone who has injured a patient because of medical negligence.

State medical boards can revoke a doctor's license if the doctor has been accused of improperly prescribing narcotic medications or other medications. For example, if your doctor has been accused of over prescribing narcotic medications to patients and if these patients have either died or have had to be admitted to hospitals, your doctor may not be allowed to practice. You need to know if your health-care provider has ever had his or her license suspended or revoked. A doctor may have practiced in another state, and lost his or her license there. Sometimes that individual will apply for a license in other states. If he or she is able to obtain a license, the doctor will move to that state. You, therefore, need to know if your health-care provider has ever had a suspended or revoked license anywhere. Some practitioners have been suspended from practicing because they were taking drugs. However, most individuals are able to return back to their respective health-care practice after going through a rehabilitation program. You should not hesitate asking what your health-care provider's grades were.

The institution that your pain-management specialist attended should also be considered. You, furthermore, need to know whether your health-care provider has had any gaps in his or her education. In other words, was he or she in school for continuous education or was his or her education interrupted. For example, if you review your health-care provider's curriculum vitae, you may note that that individual started school in 1992. If that individual was in a four-year program and did not finish until 1999, that individual has a gap in education. You should not be embarrassed to ask why. Some individuals have to interrupt their education because of money or because they had to fulfill military obligations. Other individuals may have had drug problems or personal family problems.

Furthermore, they may have had some problem in doing the course work. If you detect a gap in an individual's education, ask why there is that gap. You should also examine a curriculum vitae for the dates of each doctor that your health-care provider held. Are they chiefs of their departments? On the other hand, were they fired repetitively from positions? Health-care providers who are repeatedly dismissed from positions may have had problems with their patients or with their peers. Examine your health-care provider's curriculum vitae to see how many positions that individual has held. You may discover that your health-care provider may have been a medical director of a pain center somewhere or was head of a physical therapy or occupational therapy department. Your chiropractor may have practiced at a pain center. Your psychologist, for example, may have been on staff at a multidisciplinary pain center. Review the positions that your potential health-care provider may have had.

This information may provide you with a comfort level because you need to remember that you may have a long-term relationship with this individual. You need to know what titles your health-care provider held as well. For example, was your health-care provider a chief of pain research at a reputable institution? On the other hand, was your massage therapist a cook at a fast-food restaurant? You need to inquire about the duties of each individual about the position that they held. Did these individuals actually have hands-on relationships with their patients?

Teaching at medical schools usually involves more expertise than non-teaching professionals. Ask your health-care provider if he or she taught at any educational facility. You need to know where and when they did teach. If your pain-care provider taught anatomy at a reputable university medical school, this individual should be an expert in doing nerve blocks. This individual can also be an expert in determining what anatomic site is the cause of your pain. Check the curriculum vitae or ask your health-care provider if he or she has been on the faculty of any seminars, conferences, or workshops.

Again, someone who has recognition in his or her field is usually asked to be a faculty member at a local or national seminar or local or nation conference. Some individuals are asked to help with workshops. Workshops are hands-on teaching experiences for health-care providers. For example, pain-medicine doctors can go to a workshop to learn how to do radiofrequency ablation of nerves in facet joints. These are hands-on courses with faculty who are well experienced in these procedures. Did your health-care provider speak on reflex sympathetic dystrophy or post-herpetic neuralgia? The subject matter they spoke on usually indicates that they have some expertise in these particular fields. If you have a certain pain syndrome, you will probably want to go to an individual who has special expertise in treating this syndrome.

If you have been injured on the job or have been injured in a motor-vehicle accident or in a fall in a store, it is helpful to know if your health-care provider usually sees patients referred by insurance companies, by attorneys, or by other doctors. If you have obtained a bodily injury, you may think that discovering this information is ridiculous. However, many doctors have their referrals primarily from insurance companies. If this happens, there is the chance that bias could be introduced into your pain management.

For example, if you sustained a RSD/CRPS injury in the course of your employment, your employer may want to send you to a doctor who they routinely use for their examinations. Furthermore, a workmen's compensation insurance company may want you to see one of their doctors. Unfortunately, in some instances the company wants you to see a health-care provider who will find nothing wrong with you. This is an instance where bias is introduced into pain management. If a doctor consistently finds objective evidence to substantiate an employee's pain, that doctor may not be referred to again by the insurance company. These health-care providers are rare, but they do exist. So beware! You should, therefore, ask your potential health-care provider if he or she sees a significant number of patients referred by insurance companies.

You may have family or friends who have gone to a particular health-care provider, whether it was a chiropractor or doctor, who has significantly helped their pain. Remember that each individual has different reasons for their pain. For example, if you have read the chapter in this book on RSD/CRPS, you realize that there are many causes for RSD/CRPS pain. Your friend's chiropractor can provide significant relief for him or her if he or she has a misalignment of the knee. However, if you are suffering from osteoporosis from RSD/CRPS and have a significant loss of bone density, chiropractic may not provide you with any relief. If you have significant osteoporosis, you may ultimately need care by a rheumatologist or an endocrinologist.

In most phonebooks, you will notice advertisements for pain management. Health-care providers throughout the advertising section of a telephone book will tout their expertise in treating your pain. Chiropractors, podiatrists, anesthesiologists, neurologists, physical medicine and rehabilitation specialists, psychologists, and acupuncturists can all tell you that they will help you with your pain syndrome. The question remains, can they? It is assumed that you will not buy a new or used vehicle without researching the pros and cons of purchasing that particular vehicle. You do this research because purchasing that vehicle can be expensive.

 However, you also need to realize that pain management can be expensive. Insurance plans cover only so many procedures and types of procedures. You need to know that not every procedure is covered under a particular insurance plan. Insurance companies usually only cover methods that have been demonstrated by evidence-based medicine to be reliable and therapeutic and not dangerous. You should talk to your customer service representative at your insurance company before choosing a pain-management provider.

If you choose the wrong health-care provider for your particular condition, you can spend enormous sums of money only to find out that you will experience no pain relief. The problem is that most individuals who experience severe pain are looking for some hope that they can escape this pain. If that individual just sees an ad where his or her pain will be totally relieved, he or she becomes excited and rushes to that health-care provider. If you anticipate that you will go to court, you will want someone who has testified 50 percent for an insurance company and 50 percent for their patients. This information usually indicates to a jury or judge that your health-care provider is not biased. It may also indicate to you that you will not be undertreated or overtreated.

Because there are no real state or federal requirements for an individual to be a pain-management provider, you are ultimately responsible for choosing the correct individual. It is also important to know if your health-care provider did publish articles, book chapters, or reviews on certain pain conditions that you may be experiencing. More specifically, did your health-care provider research and do an article on your particular pain syndrome? Advertisements are not the place to discover new revolutionary treatments. Remember that if this particular treatment was safe and efficacious, the local university pain center would be utilizing this procedure.

If you are in doubt about the efficacy of a procedure, do not hesitate calling a university pain center to see whether anyone has heard of the procedure and if they recommend the procedure. You should begin to see that you are going to need to have some involvement in choosing the right care giver for your particular pain syndrome. You should not be misled by false claims from sometimes unscrupulous practitioners. Unfortunately, health care is a business like any other business. This is the reason why you need to find a health-care practitioner who is knowledgeable as well as ethical.

You also need to know whether your health-care provider has obtained certifications, titles, or designations that in effect he or she purchased and did not truly earn. Unfortunately, health-care providers can attend no courses, take no tests, or obtain designations by being "grandfathered in." An unethical health-care provider will leave unearned credits off of their curriculum vitae. In other words, did your psychologist actually earn a doctorate in psychology or was it given to that individual for life experience? You need to know what professional organizations and societies that your health-care provider is a member of.

You need to know what their status is in these organizations. If you are a cancer patient, for example, you may want to go to a health-care provider who is a member of the American Cancer Society. The problem with pain syndromes is that most pain syndromes do not fall into categories that usually can be treated by one specialist. Patients who have complex pain problems such as RSD/CRPS patients sometimes require the skills of several health-care providers to manage their pain. Pain-management techniques are now being taught in some medical schools. It is anticipated that this training will increase at least to where medical students can take an elective in pain medicine.

Hopefully some day pain medicine will become a separate specialty that is recognized as a true specialty by the American Medical Association. It is unreasonable to expect one individual to know and comprehend the entire range of knowledge associated with pain medicine without extra training in pain medicine. This is the reason why a multidisciplinary approach to pain management has evolved. This type of approach utilizes the expertise of various disciplines that are brought together in an effort to provide you with optimum pain management care.

You must do your homework when evaluating any method for pain-relieving medicines and devices sold over the counter that range from scientific nonsense to fraud. Some physicians will include testimonials from patients in their advertisements. There is no way of knowing whether these individuals actually exist. Testimonials can be a marketing tool not only for health-care products but for almost any type of product. Most of the time, you can take the testimonials that appear in advertisements with a grain of salt. If you are evaluating a medicine or a product, look for studies on the Internet or in your library.

23. Sympathetic Injections

Sympathetic injections are sometimes used to treat RSD/CRPS pain. If sympathetic injections provide pain relief then the RSD is called sympathetic maintained pain. Further sympathetic blocks can provide you with pain relief. If a sympathetic block provides no pain relief, your pain is called sympathetically independent pain and no further sympathetic blocks are necessary. If you have sympathetically maintained pain, injections should be initiated 12-16 weeks from the onset of your symptoms to be effective.

In order to understand how sympathetic injections work and how each is done, you must have some knowledge of your sympathetic nervous system. The sympathetic and the parasympathetic nervous system are parts of what is commonly called the autonomic nervous system (ANS). Autonomic means that you have no control over this nervous system. In other words, it can not be controlled by your mind. You can say that these systems should work in balance with each other and directly or indirectly affect most structures in your body (e.g. heart beat, blood pressure, blood vessels, stomach and intestines etc.). The sympathetic nervous system has an active stimulating function, while the parasympathetic has mainly a relaxing function.

The organs of our body, such as the heart, stomach and intestines, are regulated by the autonomic nervous system. The ANS is part of the peripheral nervous system and it controls many organs and muscles within your body. In most situations, we are unaware of the workings of the ANS because it functions in an involuntary, reflexive manner. For example, we do not notice when blood vessels change size or when our heart beats faster. However, some people can be trained to control some functions of the ANS such as heart rate or blood pressure with hypnosis or biofeedback. The sympathetic nervous system is located to the sympathetic chain, which connects to skin, blood vessels and organs in the body cavity. The sympathetic chain is located on both sides of the spine and consists of ganglia.

Each ganglia is composed of nerve cell bodies and exist outside of the spinal cord. The sympathetic nervous system activates what is often termed the fight or flight response. Like other parts of the nervous system, the sympathetic nervous system operates through a series of interconnected neurons. Sympathetic neurons are frequently considered part of the peripheral nervous system, although there are many neuron that lie within the central nervous system. Sympathetic neurons of the spinal cord communicate with peripheral sympathetic neurons via a series of sympathetic ganglia. Within the ganglia, spinal cord sympathetic neurons join peripheral sympathetic neurons through chemical synapses.

Spinal cord sympathetic neurons are called preganglionic neurons, while peripheral sympathetic neurons are called postganglionic neurons. At synapses within the sympathetic ganglia, preganglionic sympathetic neurons release acetylcholine, a chemical messenger that binds and activates nicotinic acetylcholine receptors on postganglionic neurons. In response to this stimulus, postganglionic neurons principally release norepinephrine. Prolonged activation of the sympathetic nervous system can elicit the release of adrenaline from the adrenal medulla. Once released, noradrenaline and adrenaline bind adrenergic receptors on peripheral tissues. Binding to adrenergic receptors causes the effects seen during the fight-or-flight response as well as the effects seen in RSD. These include pupil dilation, increased sweating, increased heart rate, and increased blood pressure.

Axons (branches that travel away from the neuron) of these nerves leave the spinal cord in the anterior (ventral) branches (rami) of the spinal nerves, and then separate out as 'white rami' which connect to two chain ganglia extending alongside the vertebral column on the left and right. These elongated ganglia are also known as paravertebral ganglia or sympathetic trunks. In these hubs, connections (synapses) are made which then distribute the nerves to major organs, glands, and other parts of the body. The ANS regulates the following: muscles in the skin (around hair follicles, smooth muscle) around blood vessels (smooth muscle) in the eye (the iris; smooth muscle) in the stomach, intestines and bladder (smooth muscle) of the heart (cardiac muscle) and some glands. Suppose you are taking a hike through the woods. You come upon a rattle snake that is coiled and is ready to strike at you. Should you stay and fight or should you turn and run? These are fight or flight responses. In these types of situations, your sympathetic nervous system becomes active. Your sympathetic nervous system increases your blood pressure and increases, your heart rate, and your digestion slows down.

Remember that your sympathetic nervous system originates in your spinal cord. In review, the cell bodies of the first neuron which we called the preganglionic neuron are located in the thoracic and lumbar spinal cord. Axons from these neurons project to a chain of ganglia located near the spinal cord. In most cases, this neuron makes a connection with another neuron (postganglionic neuron) in the ganglion. A few preganglionic neurons go to other ganglia outside of the sympathetic chain and synapse there. These postganglionic neurons then project to either a muscle or a gland.

You need to be aware that the connections between nerves in the sympathetic ganglion uses acetylcholine as a neurotransmitter. The synapse of the post-ganglionic neuron with the target organ uses the neurotransmitter called norepinephrine. (Of course, there is one exception: the sympathetic post-ganglionic neuron that terminates on the sweat glands uses acetylcholine.) The enteric nervous system is a third division of the autonomic nervous system that you do not hear much about. The enteric nervous system is a meshwork of nerve fibers that innervate the viscera (gastrointestinal tract, pancreas, and gall bladder). You can get RSD like pain in your abdomen referred to as abdominal hyperalgesia.

The cell bodies of the parasympathetic nervous system are located in the spinal cord (sacral region) and in the medulla. In the medulla, the cranial nerves III, VII, IX and X form the preganglionic parasympathetic fibers. The preganglionic fiber from the medulla or spinal cord projects to ganglia very close to the target organ and makes a synapse. This synapse uses the neurotransmitter called acetylcholine. From this ganglion, the post-ganglionic neuron projects to the target organ and uses acetylcholine again at its terminal.

As previously stated in this chapter, the stellate ganglion refers to the ganglion formed by the fusion of the inferior cervical and the first thoracic ganglion as they meet in front of the vertebral body of the seventh cervical vertebral body (C7). The structures anterior to the ganglion include the skin and subcutaneous tissue, the sternocleidomastoid, and the carotid sheath. The dome of the lung lies in front of and below the ganglion. The prevertebral fascia, vertebral body of C7, your esophagus, and your thoracic duct lie toward the center of your neck. Structures behind your ganglion include the longus colli muscle, anterior scalene muscle, vertebral artery, brachial plexus sheath, and the neck of your first rib.

You will be placed on your back with your neck placed slightly backward. Your the head will be rotated slightly to the side opposite the block. You will be asked to keep your jaw open during the injection. The point of needle puncture is located between your trachea and your carotid artery sheath at the level of your cricoid cartilage and your sixth cervical vertebra. Although the ganglion lies at the level of the C7 vertebral body, the needle is inserted at the level of C6 to avoid the piercing your lung which could cause you a breathing problem. Your neck will be washed with a surgical soap before your injection to prevent an infection and a drape will be placed over your neck. Skin anesthesia is obtained with a skin wheal of local anesthetic like lidocaine. The neck (sternocleidomastoid) muscle and your carotid artery are retracted laterally as the index and middle fingers locate a part of your sixth cervical vertebra. The skin and subcutaneous tissue are pressed firmly onto the bone to reduce the distance between the skin surface and your bone. This maneuver will push your of the your lung out of the path of the needle.

The needle is directed onto the bone and then redirected medially and downward toward the body of C6. After the bone is contacted, the needle is withdrawn 1-2 mm. This brings the needle out of the belly of the longus colli muscle which sits posterior to the ganglion and runs along the anterolateral surface of the cervical neck bones. The needle is then held immobile. The needle position is subsequently confirmed by X ray. The spread of the X ray dye is confirmed by both vertical and horizontal X ray views. Failure of the solution to spread upwards and downwards between tissue planes suggests an injection into the longus colli muscle. Immediate disappearance of the injection indicates an injection into one of your blood vessels.

A 10 cc syringe filled with a local anesthetic is attached to the needle and aspiration is performed to rule-out blood vessel placement. A 0.5 cc test dose is performed to rule out blood vessel injection into your vertebral artery. The usefulness of this test dose to provide an early warning of artery injection. This is important because seizures can occur immediately after injection even with very small volumes of local anesthetic. This test dose is followed by a 3 ml epinephrine-containing test dose to rule-out intravenous placement. The remainder of the anesthetic is injected in divided doses of 3 ml with intermittent aspiration to insure that the needle tip has not moved. Because of the risks involved with this procedure, you should have it done by a trained Board Certified Pain physician. Complications can be minimized by using an X ray machine. As with any procedure, complications can occur. You can have bruising of your skin, nerve injury, lung collapse, esophageal perforation, seizures, death, a spinal block with temporary total body paralysis, hoarseness. an elevated hemidiaphragm, infection and meningitis.

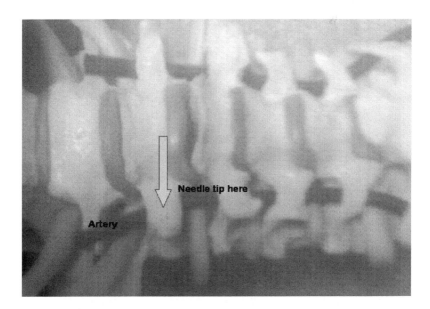

Figure 1. The arrow tip corresponds to the desired placement of the needle for a stellate ganglion block. The neck in this picture is a sideways position and the head is to the right of the picture, while the lungs are to the left of the figure. Note the position of the artery. Your doctor wants

Another type of sympathetic block is the lumbar sympathetic block. This injection is done for the treatment of RSD pain of your leg. Lumbar Sympathetic Block is an injection of local anesthetic in the "sympathetic nerve tissue" - the nerves which are a part of the Sympathetic Nervous System. The nerves are located in the back, on the either side of spine. The Lumbar sympathetic injection blocks the sympathetic nerves that go to your legs.

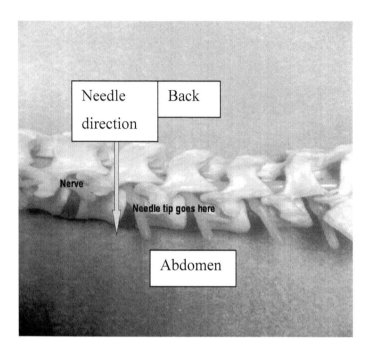

Figure 2. When you have a lumbar sympathetic block you are placed face down on your abdomen. The needle is advanced just anterior to your back bone. Your head direction is located to the left of the arrow.

Remember that the stellate ganglion injection blocks sympathetic nerves which go to your arms. This may in turn reduce pain, swelling, color abnormalities, and sweating changes in your upper or lower extremity (depending on which block is performed) and may improve pain, stiffness and improve mobility. It is done as a part of the treatment of reflex sympathetic dystrophy. herpes zoster (shingles) involving your lower extremities, vascular insufficiency and peripheral neuropathy.

Both the stellate and lumbar sympathetic injections take only a few minute to do. The block consists of a local anesthetic like lidocaine or bupiva-caine, epinephrine adrenaline and in some cases, steroids. Each injection involves inserting a needle through your skin and deeper tissues just like a flu shot. There is only minimal discomfort involved. However, most doctors numb the skin and deep tissues with a local anesthetic using a very thin needle. The block needle itself is very thin as well. before inserting the actual block needle. There is no reason for you to be unconsciousness for any of these procedures.

Each procedure is done under local anesthesia. If you request, each procedure can be done after you receive a pill like Valium given by mouth that is sedating, and this medication will make each procedure easier to tolerate. Unlike the stellate ganglion block, the lumbar sympathetic block is performed with you in the face down position. You will be monitored with a heart monitor, a blood pressure cuff and a blood oxygen-monitoring device called a pulse oximeter. Temperature sensing probes may also be placed on your hands or feet. The skin on your back is cleaned with a surgical antiseptic solution and then the injection is done. X-rays are used to guide the needle to the proper position.

You should have a ride home after the injection. I advise patients to take it easy for a day or so after their procedures. Perform the activities as tolerated by you. Some of the patients may go for immediate physical therapy. Immediately after the stellate ganglion block or the lumbar sympathetic block, you may feel your upper or lower extremities becoming warm. In addition, you may notice that your pain may be less. Unless there are complications, you should be able to return to your work the next day. The most common thing you may feel is soreness in the neck at the injection site. The local anesthetic wears off in a few hours. However, the blockade of sympathetic nerves may last for many more hours, days or weeks.

Usually, the duration of relief gets longer after each injection. If you respond to the first injection, you will be recommended for repeat injections. Usually, a series of such injections is needed to treat the problem. Some patients may need only 2 to 4 injections and some may need more than 10. The response to such injections varies from patient to patient. It is very difficult to predict if the injection(s) will help you or not.

The patients who present early for injections during their illness tend to respond better than those who have this treatment after about six months of symptoms. Patients in the advanced stages of disease may not respond adequately. These procedures are safe. However, with any procedure there are risks, side effects, and possibility of complications. The most common side effect is pain after the injection which is temporary. The other risk involves bleeding, infection, spinal block causing spinal paralysis, epidural block, and injection of the local anesthetics directly into blood vessels (seizure, arrhythmias or cardiac arrest) and surrounding organs.

Fortunately, the serious side effects and complications are uncommon. If you are allergic to any of the medications to be injected, if you are on blood thinning medications (e.g. Coumadin®, Plavix®, Ticlid®), or if you have an active infection going on near the injection site, you should not have the injection.

24. Electrical Stimulation

Pain relief may be obtained by electrical current and is now based on transcutaneous or percutaneous nerve stimulation, deep stimulation, posterior spinal cord stimulation, and transcutaneous cranial stimulation. Transcutaneous electrical nerve stimulation (TENS) is effective in controlling pain associated with RSD/CRPS. Transcutaneous electrical nerve stimulation however, is only effective if it acts on neurogenic pain/neuropathic pain, only if the nerve pathways to be stimulated are superficial and only if the conduction pathways between the area of stimulation and the superior centers are intact.

The most common form of electrical stimulation used for pain control is the transcutaneous electrical nerve stimulation (TENS) therapy, which provides short-term pain relief. Electrical nerve stimulation and electro-thermal therapy are used to relieve pain associated with various conditions. TENS is the acronym for Transcutaneous Electrical Nerve Stimulation. A TENS unit is a pocket size portable, battery-operated device that sends electrical impulses to certain parts of the body to inter-fere with pain signals going to your brain.

The electrical currents produced are mild, but can prevent pain messages from being transmitted to the brain and may raise the level of endorphins (natural pain killers produced by the brain). A TENS unit is sometimes of value in an effort to break the pain cycle. Adhesive patches which are electrodes are attached to your skin, and small electrical impulses are delivered to underlying nerve fibers. This works in two ways.

The first is through endorphins. The body has its own mechanisms for suppressing pain. Your body releases natural chemicals called endorphins in your brain, which act as pain relieving substances. TENS units can activate this mechanism. Secondly, the electrical stimulation of the nerve fibers through the electrodes can actually block a pain signal from being carried all the way to the brain. If it is blocked, the pain is not felt. Patients who use TENS units may experience significant pain relief, while at the same time engaging in a therapy that is drug-free.

TENS units have not helped significantly with all cases of RSD/CRPS because the electrode placement is difficult and there is no carryover relief from TENS treatment which means that when the unit is turned off, the pain comes back Treatment is directed at the relief of pain so the patient can begin more progressive rehabilitation caused by the disease itself. Stimulation of the spinal cord and nerve endings by electrical current is done to relieve pain. when the unit is turned off, the pain comes back

Interferential stimulation which is another form of electrical therapy and has been used for pain relief and has the benefit of extending relief post-treatment. Because the units are large, expensive, and require greater amounts of electrical energy, the patient would have to go to a facility for treatments. There are some interferential units that are portable and are powered by an AC adapter or by batteries for home use. The patient can self treat as needed. The carryover relief period seems to extend for longer periods of time as more treatments are done.

Interferential current therapy involves the placement of two electrodes on the skin at a painful area or the spinal nerve root associated with a painful region. Alternating currents of medium frequency are applied through the electrodes to the area. The currents rise and fall at different frequencies. It is theorized that the low frequency of the interferential current causes inhibition or habituation of the nervous system, which results in muscle relaxation, suppression of pain and acceleration of healing. uses a medium-frequency of alternating currents to incite tissues of injured muscles and joints.

The medium-frequency is carried by the two independent circuits of paired electrodes. Interferential stimulation is believed to reduce pain, decrease swelling or edema in tissues and increases blood circulation in damaged tissues, thus stimulating repair and health. RSD/CRPS can cause decreased blood flow in affected muscles. This modality may provide some relief. Treatments using neuromuscular stimulators on the other hand, create involuntary muscle contractions that minimize the degenerative changes in muscles that usually occur following immobilization or partial denervation. Neuromuscular Stimulation is indicated for use in conditions that may result in disuse atrophy (muscle wasting) These devices can be combined with TENS units as well (Figure 1).

Electronic Muscle Stimulation is called EMS. This type of electrical stimulation is characterized by a low volt stimulation targeted to stimulate motor nerves to cause a muscle contraction. Contraction/relaxation of muscles has been found to effectively treat a variety of musculoskeletal and vascular conditions. Most common uses of EMS are to prevent or retard disuse atrophy, strengthening programs, reeducation of muscles and reduction of muscle spasms. EMS differs from TENS in that it is designed to stimulate muscle motor nerves, while TENS is designed to stimulate sensory nerve endings to help decrease pain.

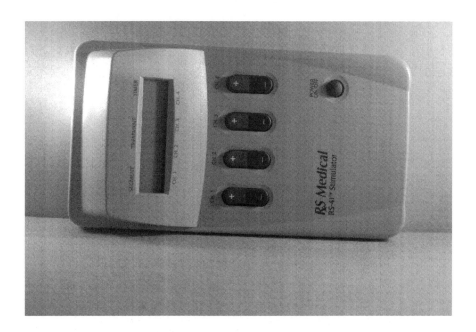

Figure 1. This is a combination TENS/muscle stimulator. It is useful in restoring muscle mass caused by lack of use if muscles in an arm or leg affected by CRPS.

If all treatments fail, implantation of a dorsal column stimulator may provide pain relief for patients suffering from RSD/CRPS. A trial electrode is placed initially. You will then assess the efficacy of the electrical stimulation. If you receive more than 50% pain relief, you will be a candidate for surgical implantation of both the battery as well as he stimulator lead wire.

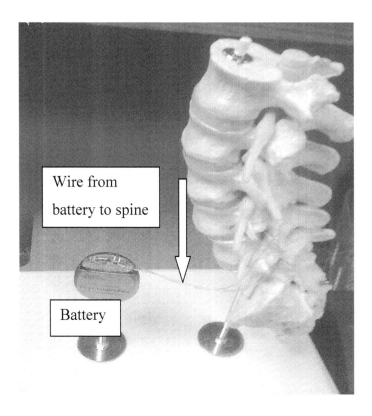

Wire from
battery to spine

Battery

Figure 2. The battery is on the left side of the picture. A wire connects the battery to the spinal cord lead in your spine.

Spinal cord stimulators are surgically implanted devices which are designed to provide pain relief from chronic intractable pain. Prior to placing an implantable spinal cord stimulator, typically the patients receives a trial of a temporary stimulator to assess the efficacy of stimulation in providing pain relief for that patient. The surgical procedure involves placing a compact generator in the lower anterior abdomen wall and connecting a wire to a strip of electrodes placed adjacent to the back part of the spinal cord. Through low-voltage electrical stimulation of the electrodes, the normal pain signals which travel in the posterior parts of the spinal cord are altered to provide partial or complete pain relief from conditions such as cancer pain, post-spinal cord injury pain, and pain from reflex sympathetic dystrophy (RSD/CRPS).

Modern spinal cord stimulators are programmable so that once implanted, the signal can be adjusted for optimal pain relief. All neurostimulation systems use low intensity electrical impulses to keep the pain signals from reaching the brain. These electrical impulses produce a tingling or massaging sensation known as paresthesia. When patients are selected carefully and the systems' electrodes are positioned properly, neurostimulation can be a successful therapy for certain types of neuropathic pain.

Neurostimulation systems typically consist of three components designed to work together:1. Leads are very thin cables, or wires, with small electrodes that deliver the electrical impulses to the nerves. 2. The generator is the power source that sends electrical energy to the electrodes. 3. The programmer allows the patient to change programs and turn the stimulation up or down. Three types of neurostimulation systems are used: radio-frequency (RF), conventional implantable pulse generator (IPG), or rechargeable IPG systems. The use of radiofrequency systems which utilize an outside battery has decreased dramatically since the introduction of rechargeable technology.

The merits of the systems are often debated, and the efficacy of each can vary from one patient to another, from one body area to another, and from one disease state to another. Additionally, research is still needed to determine whether incisions made when implanting the system can result in the spread of RSD/CRPS to other parts of the body. RSD/CRPS is sometimes a migrating or progressive disease: pain may begin in one area or extremity, only to spread and involve other extremities. This progression can significantly increase the power and electrode requirements for RSD/CRPS patients. Patients also should be aware that, because the systems contain metal, if they receive an implanted system, they cannot be exposed to magnetic resonance imaging (MRI).

Pain relief with SCS appears to decrease over time. Despite the diminishing effectiveness of SCS over time, 95% of patients with an implant would repeat the treatment for the same result. Although life-threatening complications with SCS are rare, other adverse events are frequent. On average, 34% of patients who received a stimulator had an adverse occurrence. The finding of SCS being both more effective and less expensive as compared with the standard treatment protocol for chronic RSD/CRPS renders SCS a superior technology to other RSD/CRPS treatments, meaning that there is compelling evidence for its adoption and appropriate utilization. In order to have success with a spinal cord stimulator for the management of RSD/CRPS pain, careful patient selection must be made.

The proportion of patients with intractable pain successfully managed with spinal cord stimulation however, remains disputed by some investigators. Pain reduction was sustained in those patients who continued to use the stimulator for several years. Most patients who received a dorsal column stimulator would choose to receive in an electrical stimulator again. Normalization or improvement in Quantitative Sudomotor Axon Reflex Tests and thermography have been documented in the patients with RSD who received stimulators. A rigid selection protocol can maximize the proportion of patients with intractable pain who are successfully treated with SCS. Strict neurosurgical technique eliminates infection risk. Hardware selection minimizes the incidence of malfunction.

In summary, electrical modalities can be very effective in the management of RSD/CRPS.

25. RSD/CRPS in Elderly Patients

RSD/CRPS is not uncommon in elderly patients (65 years and over). It may occur following a stroke, heart attack, bone fractures etc. Elderly patients react differently to treatments than younger patients. Pain management in general in elderly patients can be a challenge. Elderly patients can be taking many different medications. Some of these drugs can adversely interact with some pain medications. Senile patients may forget to take their medications as prescribed. Their kidneys do not function as well as in younger patients. Your kidneys are responsible for eliminating drugs. As a result, drugs like morphine can accumulate within an elderly patient's body which could cause an overdose.

Your liver metabolizes (breaks down drugs). Liver function decreases with age. An elderly patient's body mass may be decreased as well. As a result, there is less body volume where a drug can go. A dose of drug will be distributed through various body tissues. If you are emaciated, a dose of drug will remain in your blood stream instead of being distributed throughout your body. As a result, the concentration of drug in your blood stream may be higher than expected.

With respect to pain management, older patients handle pain medications differently than younger patients. Your kidneys become smaller with age. As a result, there is decreased blood flow to the kidney and less effective filtration with removal of a drug from the kidney. As one ages, the liver undergoes a decrease in mass and blood flow. Decreased saliva noted in some older patients may interfere with swallowing. Drugs prescribed by mouth may be absorbed differently because of changes in stomach acid levels in older patients. The changes in physiology with aging may alter the side effect profile of many drugs.

Depression is common in older patients. Inactivity can lead to deconditioning. Many elderly patients take pain for granted and do not mention it unless they are asked. The assessment of patients with impaired cognition may be challenging. Patients with dementia may be able to describe their current symptoms but unable to reliably report their previous symptoms.

Depression, secondary gain, personality disorders, and psychologic stress should be evaluated in all elderly patients.

The patient's physical examination should focus on the musculoskeletal system and include palpation for trigger points, evaluation for joint swelling and inflammation, and evaluation for pain with passive range of motion. Pain is suggested by facial grimacing, frowning, or repetitive eye blinking. In the elderly, pain often has multiple causes, and no single predominant cause can be identified. Poor pain management decreases the patient's quality of life and may contribute to suicide. The elderly are more likely than younger patients to experience adverse effects of analgesics. Drug dosing starting low and going upward slowly. Oral analgesic administration is usually preferred because it is convenient and results in relatively steady blood levels.

Acetaminophen is the analgesic of choice for most elderly people with mild to moderate pain. Despite its relative lack of anti-inflammatory activity, acetaminophen is usually the best drug for initial treatment of osteoarthritis. NSAIDs are indicated when inflammation contributes significantly to pain. Adverse effects vary, and a patient may tolerate one NSAID better than another. NSAIDs tend to have a ceiling analgesic dose which means that more medicine will not result in greater pain relief. The most common adverse effect of all NSAIDs is gastrointestinal upset, which may require stopping the drug. Ulceration and GI bleeding can occur. Ulceration with or without bleeding can occur simultaneously or independently of each other.

The risk of ulcers and GI bleeding for people 65 years or over is 3 to 4 times higher than that for middle-aged people. NSAIDs can impair renal function and cause sodium and water retention; they should be used cautiously in the elderly, particularly in those who have a renal disorder. Nonacetylated salicylates may have less renal toxicity and fewer antiplatelet effects than other NSAIDs.

Opioids are the most potent analgesics. Opioids act by blocking receptors in the brain and spinal cord. In the elderly, opioids have an increased half-life and possibly a greater analgesic effect than in younger patients. Nonetheless, the most common error in prescribing these drugs is to give them too infrequently, allowing breakthrough pain. A few opioids have specific advantages and disadvantages in elderly patients. Fentanyl in a patch form causes less histamine release and thus less vasodilation and hypotension. Meperidine should be avoided in elderly patients. Meperidine is less effective when given orally and can cause confusion; also, it is metabolized to an active form that tends to accumulate and thus may lead to central nervous system excitement and seizures.

Opioid agonist-antagonists, which have both agonist and antagonist effects on opiate receptors, often have psychotomimetic effects in the elderly. For this reason, pentazocine (Talwin) and butorphanol (Stadol) are rarely appropriate for the elderly patient. The analgesic effect of propoxyphene (Darvon) is similar to that of aspirin or acetaminophen, but dependency and renal impairment may occur. As a result, propoxyphene should not be used in the elderly patient. In patients with renal insufficiency, excretion of morphine and codeine may be delayed, resulting in undesira-bly long therapeutic or adverse effects, particularly with sustained-release formulations. In these patients, hydromorphone or oxycodone is less likely to accumulate and may be preferred.

Unlike NSAIDS, opioids have no ceiling analgesic effect as dosage is increased. The maximum dose is whatever is needed to relieve pain. However, adverse effects may limit the maximum dose that is used. Opioids cause dose-related sedation and respiratory depression. Most elderly patients taking opioids should not drive and should take precautions to prevent falls. Opioids may cause confusion. If confusion is due to an opioid, pupils are usually very constricted. Sometimes decreasing the dose may relieve confusion without significantly decreasing analgesia.

If this approach is ineffective, a different analgesic may be necessary. Opioids almost always cause constipation or urinary retention. Patients do not develop tolerance to these adverse effects. When an opioid is prescribeed, the patient's intake of fluid and fiber should be increased to try to prevent constipation. If a laxative is needed, a fiber laxative may be used. Gabapentin (Neurontin) is frequently prescribed in elderly patients. Dose reductions of gabapentin are recommended in patients with renal insufficiency. Dizziness and drowsiness are common adverse effects. Pregabilin (Lyrica) is frequently in elderly patients with post herpetic neuralgia.

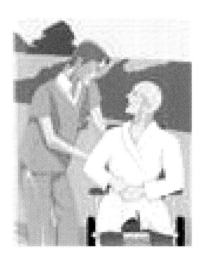

Figure 1. Pain management in an elderly patient can be a challenge.

Antidepressant medications are also prescribed as adjunct medications for elderly patients who suffer from pain. The analgesic mechanism of antidepressants ly involves interruption of brain mechanisms mediated by norepinephrine and serotonin. For tricyclic antidepressants, there is little evidence that one is better than another; however, amitriptyline, which is highly sedating and anticholinergic, should be avoided in the elderly.

Physical therapy can reduce pain due to musculoskeletal disorders in elderly patients. Aquatic therapy can help muscle and joint pain. Pain due to muscle spasm may be reduced by stretching, muscle massages, cold therapy or heat therapy. Ultrasound therapy may relieve musculoskeletal pain originating in your deep tissues. Transcutaneous electrical nerve stimulation (TENS) can relieve many types of pain as well. Alternative therapies are also used by many patients to control their pain. Occupational therapy can be helpful as well as this modality can teach patients energy saving techniques to be used around their residences.

Elderly patients can have a pronounced effect to sympathetic blocks. In other words, a patient's blood pressure can significantly drop and stellate ganglion blocks can not only decrease an elderly patient's blood pressure but can also dangerously decrease the heart rate. These procedures may need to be performed in an surgical outpatient setting where close monitoring of the patient may be accomplished.

In summary, RSD/CRPS pain management can be challenging in elderly patients. A well rained individual should be the one to treat an elderly patient.

26. RSD/CRPS in Children

Reflex sympathetic dystrophy in children is more common, and more debilitating, than many people think. Although there have been no large-scale studies on the incidence of RSD/CRPS in children, some generalizations can be made about the children who get this condition. The incidence of RSD/CRPS increases dramatically between 9 and 11 years old, and it is found predominantly in young girls. Children will fall into several diagnostic groups.

First are those who are permanently cured by treatment. The second is a group of children whose conditions are improved, but then show a high recurrence of RSD/CRPS. Fortunately each subsequence occurrence of RSD/CRPS seems less severe. A third and relatively small group of children with RSD/CRPS get progressively worse despite treatment and require aggressive intervention, even sympathectomy. A high percentage of children will improve with active mobilization of the affected extremity and psycho-social conditioning alone.

A previous published study indicated that a physician needs to remain vigilant for a recurrence of RSD/CRPS when a child goes into remission following a bout with RSD/CRPS. In that study, recurrent episodes of RSD/CRPS in children occurred in up to 40% of patients, however, most of these recurrent episodes were milder than the initial episode. The prognosis of RSD/CRPS in the children is excellent. This is due to the surge of growth hormone, endorphins, sex hormones, and other hormones during adolescence which afford the body with excellent control of healing with respect to the sympathetic system. In this age group it is rare to see a child progress to stage III. Even sympathectomy, which practically universally fails in adults with RSD/CRPS, is helpful in young patients.

Not all patients with RSD/CRPS move from stage to stage in an orderly progression, especially not children. Stage one is called the acute stage. The child's onset of RSD/CRPS may occur immediately after the initial injury or may not occur until several weeks after the event. Either way, the child experiences pain that is out of proportion to the injury. A child may have swelling (i.e., edema), redness or inflammation of the skin (i.e., erythema) and in-creased warmth; however, some children initially may have a cool extremity. Stage two is called the dystrophic stage and typically occurs three to six months after symptoms begin. RSD/CRPS can markedly disable a child and depress activities of daily living.

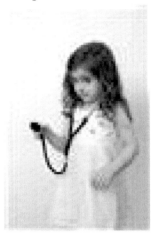

Figure 1. It is important to diagnose pediatric RSD/CRPS in a timely fashion. This disease entity can be overlooked in children.

You may notice skin and nail bed changes in your child during this stage and your child's physician may find bony demineralization by taking radiographic images. The third stage of RSD/CRPS is called the atrophic stage where a progressive decline of skin and muscle and osteopenia (i.e., a condition in which bones are not mineralized normally) can occur. Children seldom progress to the atrophic stage although stage three is not unheard of in children. Children who have RSD/CRPS type I more frequently are affected in one of their lower extremities. Children's lower extremities are affected about five times more often than upper extremities. Adults, on the other hand, are twice as likely to be affected in an upper extremity.

Most children with RSD/CRPS type I are from upper middle class families and are athletic. A typical pediatric patient with RSD/CRPS type I is a female who participates in ballet, soccer or gymnastics. Researchers have hypothesized that there may be a genetic predisposition to RSD/CRPS type I. Most children who have the syndrome are Caucasian. Treating RSD/CRPS in children typically requires a combination of anti-inflammatory medications coupled with neuropathic medications that are typically used for the treatment of pain associated with childhood diabetes. In addition, your child's pediatrician may recommend the use of physical therapy in an effort to improve the mobility and use of the arm that is affected.

When not effectively treated, RSD/CRPS can continue into adulthood and become a debilitating health condition, affecting quality of life and even causing work related disability. The key to your child's optimal health, however, will lie in early diagnosis and aggressive treatment of RSD/CRPS from not only a physical standpoint but also a mental health standpoint.

27. Facial RSD/CRPS

Facial RSD/CRPS is an infrequently reported clinical pain syndrome that presents clinicians with difficult pain evaluations and management problems. Unfortunately, sympathetically mediated orofacial pain can occur following routine tooth extraction and may not be easily recognized. Orofacial pain can be a complex entity to diagnose and treat. A problem exists in that facial reflex sympathetic dystrophy is a rare entity and is not well described in the medical or dental literature. As result, there is no consensus for treatment. The differential diagnosis of facial reflex sympathetic dystrophy includes trigeminal neuralgia, trigeminal neuropathy, glossopharyngal neuralgia and atypical facial pain. The majority of these entities can be treated with anticonvulsant and antidepressant medications.

Reflex sympathetic dystrophy of the face is frequently associated with cutaneous or inner mouth allodynia (pain to touch)that unlike trigeminal neuralgia does not follow a cranial nerve distribution. A sensory deficit may or may not be present. Tender areas are common about the face. Sweating and skin warmth or cold are less obvious in facial reflex sympathetic dystrophy than in the arms or legs. Trigeminal neuralgia, like facial reflex sympathetic dystrophy, is associated with a sensory deficit with neurologic testing. However, the pain associated with trigeminal neuralgia is in the distribution of the trigeminal nerve (upper and lower jaw)as opposed to being more global as is the case facial reflex sympathetic dystropy.

Atypical facial pain is refractory to analgesics, sympathetic nerve blocks, and surgical resection of the fifth and ninth cranial nerves. This pain may represent a behavioral disorder. The treatment of this disorder, as well as the previously mentioned facial pain disorders, can be accomplished with anti-inflammatory drugs, antidepressants, and anticonvulsants. However, in atypical facial pain, these modalities are usually unsatisfactory. The facial reflex sympathetic dystrophy treatment response to sympathetic blockade appears to be efficacious and is reported to be less dependent on timing from the time of onset of symptoms until the initiation of sympathetic blockade. In other words, facial reflex sympathetic dystrophy pain has a favorable prognosis and can be managed conservatively with a stellate ganglion block series, even when initiated as a delayed and repetitive injection series.

Trigeminal neuralgia is commonly treated with medications such as carbamazepine and baclofen. Gabapentin may be used if there is no pharmacologic response to carbamazepine or if a patient does not tolerate this anticonvulsant. A percutaneous computed tomography guided radiofrequency trigeminal rhizotomy can be used for the treatment of idiopathic trigeminal neuralgia. Neurosurgical procedures such as microvascular decompression and Gamma knife surgery may be of benefit as well.

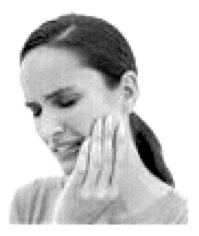

Figure 1. Facial RSD/CRPS can disable a patient. The dental profession must be aware that this entity exists and refer to a pain medicine specialist..

The pathophysiology of facial sympathetically maintained pain in laboratory studies are different than that found in peripheral nerve sympathetic models. No sprouting of sympathetic terminals occurred in the trigeminal ganglion of injured nerves as is commonly seen in the dorsal root ganglia of spinal nerves, occurring with the complex regional pain syndrome. Immunocytochemistry has been used to investigate whether autonomic fibers sprouted in the skin of the lower lip of rats in a rodent model of neuropathic pain. In order to do this study, a chronic constriction injury of a branch of the trigeminal nerve was done and calcitonin gene-related peptide (CGRP)-immunoreactive sensory fibers were identified. Sympathetic fiber sprouting was first observed one week post-injury with a peak in the number of sprouted fibers occurring at four and six weeks post-CCI.

No sympathetic fiber sprouting was noted in the trigeminal ganglion of any of the study rats following CCI. At four weeks post-CCI, the rats displayed signs of spontaneous pain. The increase in terminal sympathetic fibers apparently had a role in the generation of abnormal pain following nerve injury in this laboratory study. No temperature changes of the skin, hyperhidrosis or skin discoloration about the face or mouth were noted pre-or post-injection.

Patients with facial RSD/CRPS do not present with a typical complex regional pain syndrome seen in an extremity as defined by the International Association for the Study of Pain (IASP): the presence of regional pain and sensory changes following a noxious event, pain is associated with associated findings such as abnormal skin color, temperature change, abnormal sudomotor (sweating) activity, edema, no distribution of the pain of a single nerve in the extremity and the combination of these findings exceeds their expected magnitude in response to known physical damage during and following the inciting event.

In conclusion, the diagnosis and management of facial pain is reported to be aggravating and frustrating for patients as well as for health care providers. Patients should not be dismissed as having psychological etiologies of their pain until all potential therapeutic modalities have been assessed. Facial reflex sympathetic dystrophy is so rare that evidence-based treatment trials are essentially non-existent. It is not recommended that every patient with nonspecific post-tooth extraction pain have a stellate ganglion block. Practitioners should, however, be aware of the potential for facial reflex sympathetic dystrophy in dental related orofacial pain and make the appropriate referral for a pain medicine evaluation when other modalities have failed.

**THESE SITES MAY BE OF INTEREST TO RSD/CRPS
PATIENTS AND THEIR FAMILIES**

American Chronic Pain Association: http://www.theacpa.org

Reflex Sympathetic Dystrophy Syndrome Association:
http://www.rsds.org

American RSD Hope Organization: http://www.rsdhope.org

National Foundation for the Treatment of Pain:
http://www.paincare.org

American Pain Foundation: http://www.painfoundation.org

Mayday Fund [For Pain Research]: http://www.painandhealth.org

International Research Foundation for RSD/CRPS:
http://rsdhealthcare.org/

Index

About the Author

William E. Ackerman III, M.D., is an American Board of Anesthesiology certified anesthesiologist with American Board of Medical Specialties certification in Pain Medicine. He has over 20 years of experience in acute, chronic, cancer, intensive care and obstetric pain management. Dr. Ackerman is well published and researched in RSD/CRPS. He is a graduate of the University of Louisville School of Medicine and did his residency at the University of Kentucky. He was selected Chief Resident at the University of Kentucky when he was a senior resident in anesthesiology. He did a pain medicine fellowship at the Texas Tech University Health Sciences Center. Dr. Ackerman has an extensive academic career. Dr. Ackerman has been involved in medical research and he has presented the results of his scientific research at international and national scientific meetings. He has been a guest speaker at medical school specialty department meetings and academic symposiums throughout the country.

Dr. Ackerman has published over one hundred peer reviewed scientific articles and has published numerous book chapters in medical text-books. His books include: (1) OBSTETRIC ANESTHESIA PEARLS, (2) THE GENDER FACTOR: PAIN MANAGEMENT FOR MEN AND WOMEN (3) THE AMA GUIDES TO THE EVALUATION OF DISEASE AND INJURY CAUSATION and (4) THE PATIENT'S HANDBOOK of PAIN MANAGEMENT. He was a recipient of the Karl Koller research grant from the American Society of Regional Anesthesia and Pain Medicine. He was also nominated previously for the Southern Medical Society Research Award as well as the Bristol-Meyers Squibb Award for Distinguished Achievement in Pain Re-search. Dr. Ackerman has an extensive academic career. He has been Medical Director of Pain Medicine at the University of Arkansas for Medical Sciences. He was chief of anesthesiology at the Ireland Army Hospital at Fort Knox, Kentucky and at the William Beaumont Army Medical Center in El Paso Texas where he was involved in intern, resident and nurse anesthetist education.

He has most recently been medical director of pain medicine at the Neurosciences Center at Central Baptist Hospital in Lexington, Kentucky with an office practice and was a consultant to the hospital medical/surgical wards as well as the intensive care units. Dr. Ackerman is now in private practice and is the Medical Director of the Pain Medicine Consultants Group, PA in Little Rock, Arkansas.

Made in the USA
Lexington, KY
30 December 2013